ENDING MEDICAL REVERSAL

ENDING **MEDICAL** REVERSAL

ENDING**MEDICAL**REVƎRSAL

:: Improving Outcomes, Saving Lives

VINAYAK K. PRASAD, MD, MPH
ADAM S. CIFU, MD

JOHNS HOPKINS UNIVERSITY PRESS | Baltimore

Note to the reader: This book is not meant to substitute for medical care, and neither diagnostic decisions nor treatment should be based solely on its contents. Instead, they must be developed in a dialogue between the individual and his or her physician.

Drug dosage: The authors and publisher have made reasonable efforts to determine that the selection of drugs discussed in this text conform to the practices of the general medical community. The medications described do not necessarily have specific approval by the U.S. Food and Drug Administration for use in the diseases for which they are recommended. In view of ongoing research, changes in governmental regulation, and the constant flow of information relating to drug therapy and drug reactions, the reader is urged to check the package insert of each drug for any change in indications and dosage and for warnings and precautions. This is particularly important when the recommended agent is a new and/or infrequently used drug.

© 2015 Vinayak K. Prasad and Adam S. Cifu
All rights reserved. Published 2015
Printed in the United States of America on acid-free paper

Johns Hopkins Paperback edition, 2019
9 8 7 6 5 4 3 2 1

Johns Hopkins University Press
2715 North Charles Street
Baltimore, Maryland 21218-4363
www.press.jhu.edu

The Library of Congress has cataloged the hardcover edition of this book as follows:
Prasad, Vinayak K., 1982–, author.
    Ending medical reversal : improving outcomes, saving lives / Vinayak K. Prasad and Adam S. Cifu.
    p. ; cm.
Includes bibliographical references and index.
ISBN 978-1-4214-1772-1 (hardcover : alk. paper) — ISBN 1-4214-1772-3 (hardcover : alk. paper) — ISBN 978-1-4214-1773-8 (electronic) — ISBN 1-4214-1773-1 (electronic)
    I. Cifu, Adam S., author. II. Title.
    [DNLM: 1. Delivery of Health Care. 2. Treatment Outcome. 3. Clinical Trials as Topic. 4. Evidence-Based Medicine. 5. Therapeutics—trends. 6. Popular Works. W 84.41]
    R733
    615.5—dc23   2014049513

A catalog record for this book is available from the British Library.

ISBN-13: 978-1-4214-2904-5
ISBN-10: 1-4214-2904-7

Special discounts are available for bulk purchases of this book. For more information, please contact Special Sales at 410-516-6936 or specialsales@press.jhu.edu.

Johns Hopkins University Press uses environmentally friendly book materials, including recycled text paper that is composed of at least 30 percent post-consumer waste, whenever possible.

CONTENTS

ENDING MEDICAL REVERSAL

INTRODUCTION

THIS BOOK IS ABOUT HOW, despite tremendous advances in the clinical, genomic, and surgical sciences, doctors continue to use medical practices, sometimes for decades, that are later shown to be of no benefit to their patients. Over the past six years, we have researched and struggled with this topic, which we call *medical reversal*, and in this book we share some of our conclusions.

For those who follow the medical news, the simple fact that medical recommendations change will come as no surprise. Time and again we see enthusiasm for some medical therapy (beta carotene, vitamin E, low-fat diets) rise and fall. First there is certainty that a new practice will help extend your life, then there is equal certainty that it does not. To people outside of medicine (as well as many inside the field), this process is frustrating.

When you look at the day-to-day recommendations that doctors make—the ones that usually do not make the news—you find the story is similar. In one decade, doctors recommend an aggressive treatment of high-dose chemotherapy and stem-cell transplantation for women with breast cancer, promising that it will give a woman her best chance of a cure. Then, over the next decade, doctors report that all of that enthusiasm was misguided; the aggressive treatment was no better than a less aggressive course of therapy, which, incidentally, was what we had been doing previously.

Many people dismiss this phenomenon as the natural course of science: of course hypotheses turn out to be wrong, and we can only move forward through trial and error. Although this is certainly true in biomedical science—where there are false starts, good hypotheses that fail to live up to expectations—it is not the case in medicine. Medicine is the application of science. When a scientific theory is disproved, it should happen in a lab or in the equivalent place in clinical science, the controlled clinical trial. It should not be disproved in the world of clinical medicine, where millions of people may have already been exposed to an ineffective, or perhaps even harmful, treatment.

In this book, we hope to make the case that, when it comes to how we care for people, medicine can do a better job of recommending practices that actually work. In the long run, more and more of what doctors do can be enduring. False starts are inevitable in science, but not when we apply science to caring for people.

HISTORY

We write this book not as critical outsiders, but because, like so many other doctors, we have been there. Each of us recalls moments when we realized that what we had told our patients, or did for them, was wrong: we had promoted an accepted practice that was, at best, ineffective.

For Adam, like many doctors of his generation, the most memorable reversal was estrogen replacement for postmenopausal women. For years, he would draw the diagram in figure I.1 at least once every couple of weeks. It was a way to explain why doctors recommended that women use estrogen-replacement therapy after menopause. He would explain that the treatment would be good for the bones (decreasing the risk of osteoporosis), bad for the breasts (increasing the risk of breast cancer), and good for the heart (decreasing the risk of heart attacks). On balance, the benefits outweighed the risks. Many of his patients started the therapy.

But then a well-designed clinical trial showed that this diagram was flawed, along with the advice. Estrogen-replacement therapy was of no benefit to the heart. In fact, at least early in the course of therapy, the treatment might even carry some risk. This was a perfect example of reversal.

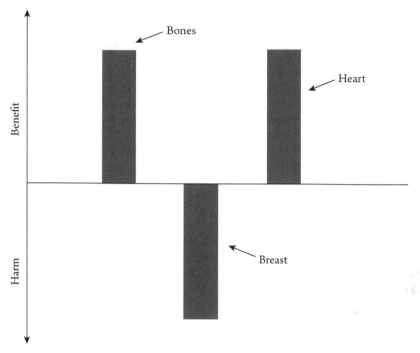

I.1 Explanation of the risks and benefits of estrogen-replacement therapy (circa 1996).

An accepted, widely used therapy was found to be ineffective or possibly harmful. Doctors stopped recommending the therapy not because we discovered something better, but because we never should have used it in the first place.

For Vinayak, the experience with reversal that resonates most occurred in the cardiac intensive care unit (CCU). It was early in his training; the hours were long and the days were grueling. There were orders to be written, tests to coordinate, medications to prescribe, ventilators to adjust, and no shortage of procedures to perform. However, when he went home each day, it was not these things that occupied his thoughts, but whether a core intervention was helping people.

For many of the patients he cared for, the CCU team would recommend placement of a coronary stent, a small, expandable, metal mesh tube that can open narrowed or blocked coronary arteries. The justification for the recommendation varied widely based on the patient's problem. For some patients, those having heart attacks, the recommendation was well-founded.

Multiple studies had shown that stents saved lives. For other patients the team recommended stents where they had not been proven effective, and in some cases, stents were recommended where they had been shown not to help. For him, the situation became tragic when one patient, who had received a stent she did not need, suffered a complication of the procedure. She experienced harm without possibility of benefit. Vinayak kept thinking, What about our oath to "do no harm"? Although we preached something called "evidence-based medicine," few of us were truly practicing it.

EVIDENCE-BASED MEDICINE AND MEDICAL REVERSAL

Twenty-five years ago, "evidence-based medicine" (EBM) was seen as the future of medicine. EBM was founded on the idea that our practice should be based on empirical evidence from studies of real patients. At its birth, EBM was revolutionary. Until that time, medical practice had been based first on hypotheses and clinical experiences and later, additionally, on our understanding of the biological underpinnings of disease. In EBM, those things were still considered important and still needed to be considered, but it was now appreciated that they should always be bolstered with information from well-done, reliable, clinical experiments.

Evidence-based medicine was accepted because of the realization that, not infrequently, practices that seemed to work and practices that the best science said should work did not. In 1981 John McKinlay, a medical sociologist, wrote an article that perfectly summarized the state of affairs in the pre-EBM world. In the article, he described the "seven stages in the career of a medical innovation." These stages began with a "promising report" in which a medical innovation is publicized based on its promise—often a good explanation of why it should work. In the second stage, the innovation is adopted by the profession, motivated by forces as disparate as belief that the innovation will benefit patients, peer pressure, and the promise of financial gain. Stage three, in which patients and payers accept the innovation as standard, follows quickly. Only at the fourth stage in McKinlay's analysis do "data" begin to enter the story. However, the data supporting the innovation come only from insubstantial studies that support the innovation in the most superficial way. (We spend a great deal of ink in this book discussing the uneven data that support medical innovations.)

Finally, at stage five, the randomized controlled trial, the foundation of evidence-based medicine, makes an appearance. This kind of reliable, experimental study may either support the innovation or prove (or at the very least suggest) that it is ineffective. The latter case is what we refer to as reversal. Stages six and seven see the response to the reliable, experimental data: first denial, as entrenched interests deny that the innovation may not be effective, and then finally acceptance.

McKinlay's article was not only brilliant but prescient as well. In writing about medicine in 1981, he addressed issues that are still with us 35 years later and made suggestions for a way forward, many of which we endorse in this book.

EBM was adopted as a way to move beyond McKinlay's seven stages. In evidence-based medicine, innovations that seemed to work and made sense would not be adopted until they were supported by robust data. By the early 1990s, EBM was becoming gospel. The *Journal of the American Medical Association* published a series of articles about how to appraise reports of clinical trials. Students were taught to dissect studies published in the medical literature. Attending physicians would hand out Xeroxed copies of articles from the week's *New England Journal of Medicine*. The most common question asked on physicians' rounds was, "What is the evidence for that?"

Over the past decade, however, the EBM revolution has not been sustained. It seems counterintuitive to say this because, by many measures, EBM is as strong as ever. We now have more evidence than ever before. Our journals are full of randomized trials and meta-analyses (combinations of randomized trials), the most reliable studies on which to base practice. We have researchers devoted to studying the evidence base of medical practice. Yet, the studies we have often avoid big questions, or they are built with so much bias—favoring one side from the start—that they are not useful. And for each practice that is shown not to work, it seems as if two more dubious ones take its place. It is not that counterrevolutionaries have seized the ramparts, but the dedication to the cause, to practicing medicine from an evidence base, has waned. Some of EBM's wane has been passive; it is hard to critically appraise every decision you, as a physician, make. Some of the wane has been less than passive, with drugmakers, device makers, and even scientists sullying the purity of the medical literature. Either way, the result has been a near epidemic of medical reversals.

What are medical reversals? We expect that medicine will progress in a generally orderly fashion, with good medical practices being replaced by better ones. We used to use cholestyramine—a horribly tolerated drug that had no effect on patients' life expectancy—to lower cholesterol after heart attacks. Now we use atorvastatin, a well-tolerated drug backed by robust evidence that it saves lives. This is how medical practice should evolve. Reversal, however, is different. Reversal occurs when a currently accepted therapy is overturned, found to be no better than the therapy it replaced. This often occurs when a practice—a diagnostic tool, a medicine, a procedure, or a surgical technique—is adopted without a robust evidence base.

In the history of medicine, the examples of reversal are legion. Books have been written about innovations that were adopted based only on a flawed theory and ended up helping no one. From medications (calomel—mercurous chloride—for the treatment of yellow fever and arsenic therapy for syphilis) to procedures (cupping—the use of topical suction to promote cure) to surgeries (lobotomy), medicine has a rich, though ignominious, history of reversals. These examples are interesting, but they are not our focus. They are treatments adopted before we had a clear path forward. We concentrate on reversals in the age of EBM, an age when we know how medicine should safely and reliably advance.

Our interest in reversal, which began during the clinical experiences that we mentioned, grew as we read article after article that overturned accepted practices. Medications that we had prescribed (estrogen replacement and rofecoxib [Vioxx]) and procedures that we had recommended (vertebroplasty, stents for stable coronary-artery disease) were among the ones overturned. We began to research the frequency, causes, and harms of reversal. The more we learned, the more we realized that not only was this a highly prevalent problem, but it was one whose solution could go a long way toward curing the ills of our health-care system. Seeing how far our field has strayed from the evidence convinced us that this was a topic that had to leave the periphery of the medical literature and enter mainstream conversations.

AUDIENCE

We write this book for people, like us, who are confused every time they see a report that a therapy that was recommended yesterday is no longer recommended today. The therapy has fallen out of favor not because it was replaced by something better but because it was found not to work (or at least not to work better than the previous standard or less invasive therapy). This news comes not only in medical journals but in newspapers, radio reports, and endless Internet coverage. In this book we give dozens of examples of medical reversal, some of which might already be familiar. We show that reversals have happened in every corner of medicine. We go to great lengths to explain the causes of reversal, the harms reversal brings, and, most importantly, possible solutions.

We propose solutions that you, and we, can use. We all have been, and will be, patients. At these times we all want to know, "How can I be sure that the treatment offered to me today will not be found wanting tomorrow?" Beyond answering this, we go further and suggest more systemic solutions that can make our field less apt to adopt tests and treatments that do not work. These solutions should be of interest to students of medicine, doctors, and policymakers.

CONTROVERSY, REFERENCES, AND PATIENTS

Some of the arguments we make in this book are controversial. We state that a sizable proportion of what doctors have done has turned out to be wrong—not wrong in retrospect but unfounded when they were doing it. We also argue that much of what doctors still do is wrong. We have made every effort in the writing of this book to steer away from controversy. When discussing practices that have been reversed, we avoid areas where there is still honest debate. Even with that care, some readers are sure to disagree with some of what we say. Sometimes, the interpretation of medical practice and scientific trials is not black and white. We hope that if you disagree with one or two of our examples or arguments, you will read on. We think that on balance, the weight of our argument will convince you.

Because of the controversy of the topic, we have tried to consider (and often offer) the other side of any debate, and we always provide references to our original sources. We list these at the end of the book, grouped by chapters. We hope you will read the ones that interest you most.

Because our work grows out of our clinical lives, we fill this book with anecdotes. All of these are composites of patients for whom we have cared. None of them is based on any single person, or even on one or two patients. Instead, they draw upon our general experience taking care of many patients.

Medicine practiced well is beautiful. As a human pursuit, it is pure—caring for the suffering. Empathy and the ability to anticipate a patient's changing needs are the hallmarks of an excellent physician. Clinical medicine can also be one of the most satisfying of intellectual pursuits. The diagnostic process and development of an effective management plan, when done well, are elegant in their thoughtfulness and parsimony. The fact that this intellectual activity is only a means to a greater end makes it even more magnificent. Conversely, medicine done poorly is painful to watch and worse to experience. It may lead to bad patient outcomes—unnecessary suffering and even death. Even practice that is only average creates anxiety for patients and doctors and runs up enormous costs to society. In the end, our goal in writing this book is to see more medicine done well and less done badly. Such a change would benefit patients, doctors, and all of us who pay for our health care.

PART 1

MEDICAL REVERSAL

:: EXAMPLES, FREQUENCY, AND CONSEQUENCES

1

WHAT IS MEDICAL REVERSAL?

WE EXPECT THAT MEDICAL THERAPY will change and evolve with time. Good treatments will replace bad ones, and then better ones will replace those. Antibiotics have replaced arsenic, and anesthesia has replaced a bullet held bracingly between the teeth. Recently, however, change has occurred in surprising ways. If you have followed the news about prostate cancer screening, mammography for women in their forties, hormone replacement, cholesterol-lowering medications, and stents for coronary-artery disease, you might think doctors cannot get anything straight. These common practices were not replaced by better therapies; they were found to be ineffective. In some cases, they did more harm than good. You might be worried that some medical practices are nothing more than fads. In some cases, you would be right.

We call this phenomenon "medical reversal." Instead of the ideal, which is replacement of good medical practices by better ones, medical reversal occurs when a currently accepted therapy is overturned—found to be no better than the therapy it replaced. Now, you might argue that this is how science is supposed to proceed. In high school, we learned that the scientific method involves proposing a hypothesis and testing to see whether it is right. This is true. But what has happened in medicine is that the hypothesized treatment is often instituted in millions of people, and billions of dollars are spent, before adequate research is done. Not surprisingly, sometimes the research demonstrates that the hypothesis was incorrect and that the treatment, which is already being used, is ineffective or harmful.

CASES OF REVERSAL

A few people's stories highlight notorious examples of reversal in medicine. Consider Samuel Jones, a 57-year-old gentleman who had a heart attack in 1991. He was admitted to the hospital and treated with the standard medical regimen, which, at the time, included flecainide, a drug used to stabilize his heart rhythm. In the late 1980s and early 1990s, flecainide and its sibling drugs were widely used with the intention of suppressing extra heartbeats (called premature ventricular contractions, or PVCs) and preventing death. The logic behind the use of these drugs was ironclad. PVCs are strongly associated with sudden death. The more you have, the more likely you are to die. And there was no better medicine for suppressing PVCs than flecainide. How could it not save lives? Some cardiologists were so confident in the drug that they would not let their patients enter studies of this medication. Such studies required that some patients be randomized to receive a placebo instead of flecainide. In all good conscience, how could they risk having their patients deprived of this lifesaving drug?

Unfortunately, flecainide did not work. In 1992, a large study called the Cardiac Arrhythmia Suppression Trial (or CAST trial) showed that flecainide, as well as a similar drug, decreased PVCs as expected but also increased patients' chance of dying.* The finding was devastating. It changed not only how we treat heart-attack patients but how we evaluate medical therapies altogether. CAST taught us that even the most careful reasoning and the best scientific models do not guarantee an effective clini-

---

* As you will see throughout this book, one of the great sports in academic medicine is to choose a name for your trial that can be reduced to a catchy, memorable acronym. In our careers we have seen not only CAST and LIFE, discussed in this chapter, but also NICE-SUGAR, CLEOPATRA, and our favorite, CABG Patch.

cal treatment. What works in the lab, or on a computer, or in the head of the smartest researcher does not always work in a patient.

But now, more than 20 years later, this is a lesson that many physicians and leading researchers still have not really learned.

Let's consider another medication, this one for high blood pressure (hypertension). Hypertension remains one of the most common ailments in America. Although most people with hypertension are entirely without symptoms, there is no doubt that hypertension strongly predicts an increased risk of stroke, heart disease, and death. It is truly a silent killer. People with naturally lower blood pressure live longer, and people who use certain medications to lower their blood pressure can decrease their risk of death. One of the first drugs used to treat hypertension was atenolol. Atenolol, a member of the beta-blocker class of antihypertensives, dramatically lowered blood pressure, and for decades it achieved the rarefied status of "trial standard," meaning that you had to show your new drug was as good as atenolol in order to get it on the market.

In 2002 something really unsettling (or maybe even terrifying) happened. After atenolol had been used to treat hypertension for nearly 20 years, the results of the LIFE trial were published. This trial compared atenolol to a newer drug, losartan. People who took losartan had fewer strokes and lived longer than those that took atenolol. At first glance it seemed that we had come up with a better antihypertensive; this seemed like an example of replacement. Somewhat surprising was that both drugs lowered blood pressure the same amount.

The question was, did losartan beat atenolol because losartan is better or because atenolol is actually ineffective? The tantalizing finding in the LIFE study was extended in 2004, when a pooled analysis of all people who took atenolol versus sugar pills (placebos) in trials showed that atenolol was no better than the placebo. Atenolol did lower people's blood pressure, but it did not decrease people's risk of dying or of having a heart attack. Let that sink in. A drug that was widely used, accepted as the standard of care, had made millions and millions of dollars for its manufacturers, and had made high blood pressure the subject of dinnertime conversation, did not make you live a single day longer. A recent study showed that metoprolol (another beta-blocker) is no better than atenolol. If you have taken a beta-blocker for high blood pressure, you may have shaved a few percentage points off your risk of stroke, but you did not extend your life. In the world of blood-pressure medicines, you took a pill that does not work.*

If the only place modern medicine erred was with medications, we would be fortunate. But there are also medical procedures, some used for decades by practitioners who have reaped huge financial rewards, that have been shown not to work.

Let's examine another person. Anthony Baker is a 55-year-old mechanic who thinks of himself as active. His job in a garage requires him to be on his feet most of the day. In the summer he mows his lawn every week—with a push mower, no less—and in the winter he shovels snow from his walk after storms. Anthony does not have any health problems—well, at least that he knows of—and he sees his doctor yearly. At his last checkup, he was told that he was in fine health, aside from the yearly advice to quit smoking.

Over the past few months, however, Anthony has noticed that when he exerts himself, he feels an ache in his chest. This "pressure" resolves after about five minutes of rest. Anthony calls his doctor to tell him about the chest tightness. His doc is concerned that Anthony might have developed coronary-artery disease and that his symptoms represent angina.

Angina is cardiac pain that occurs when the heart's demand for oxygen outstrips its supply. It often happens during exertion because that is when the demand for oxygen is greatest. Anthony's doctor orders a stress test, a test that examines the heart's function during exercise. The test shows that Anthony has a narrowing in his circumflex coronary artery (one of the three coronary arteries that supply oxygenated blood to the heart). Based on the results of the test, the doctor diagnoses Anthony with coronary-artery disease, tells him to stop smoking, starts him on a few medications (metoprolol, a beta-blocker, to lessen the heart's oxygen demand; atorvastatin, a cholesterol-lowering medication; and aspirin). He also schedules him to see a cardiologist the following week.

When Anthony sees the cardiologist, he has not yet started his medications and reports one episode of chest pain that occurred while he was walking his dog over the weekend. The cardiologist schedules Anthony for a coronary angiogram. During an angiogram dye is injected into the coronary arteries to assess their patency—to determine whether or not there

---

* We are only talking about hypertension. If you have heart failure, you really need your carvedilol or metoprolol succinate!

are blockages. The angiogram shows a 90 percent blockage of his circumflex artery. During the procedure the cardiologist places a stent, a metal tube, in the artery and the 90 percent blockage disappears. He gives Anthony another prescription, this one for clopidogrel, a blood thinner, to add to the rest of his medications.

One week later Anthony sees his regular doctor and is pleased to say that, despite having shoveled six inches of snow the previous day, he is feeling the best he has felt in years. He has no pain and, in fact, he recognizes that he was probably having more chest symptoms than he was aware of before the procedure.

So, was Anthony cured by the cardiologist? It is undeniable that Anthony feels better.* You may also be thinking that Anthony narrowly made it— that if he had not had the artery opened, he would have had a heart attack. That because of the stent, Anthony will live longer. And though the procedure cost more than $10,000, on the whole, it must be worth it.

But what if we told you that Anthony is no less likely to have a heart attack. What if we add that Anthony will not live a single day longer. And, perhaps, most concerning, what if we tell you that in 12 months, Anthony's chest pain will be the same, even though he had the stent. Did Anthony really benefit?

There is a long list of medical procedures whose use is based on scientific evidence that is, at best, suspect. Vertebroplasty is another great example. For years, doctors struggled to treat people (mostly women) who suffered osteoporotic fractures of the spine. These fractures can lead to chronic back pain. In the late 1990s, a couple of radiologists had a brilliant idea. Why not insert a needle into the fractured bone and inject medical-grade cement. The theory was that the cement would plump up the bone, the nerves would get some extra breathing room as the fractured bone was lifted away, and the pain would dissipate. When these pioneers performed the procedure, vertebroplasty, on a few dozen patients, they were amazed with the results. Patients immediately felt better. Patients and doctors were convinced.

In the very early 2000s, interested parties lobbied Medicare to pay for

---

* In later chapters we'll learn about other procedures that make people feel better but provide no real benefit. These examples will make you reconsider the whole "feeling better" issue.

vertebroplasty, and their request was granted. In a few years, tens of thousands of people were having the procedure each year. By the end of the decade, vertebroplasty was a billion-dollar-a-year industry. There were complications—rarely, the cement would go somewhere it was not supposed to—but on the whole, this procedure seemed like a real advance. In 2009 two groups of brave investigators put vertebroplasty to the true test. They enrolled 200 patients. Half of the patients got vertebroplasty; the other half were taken to the procedure room and prepped for the procedure; the cement was opened, so patients could smell it; and salt water was injected. Both groups of patients, those that got vertebroplasty and those that had a sham procedure, had identical improvements. Vertebroplasty, as it turned out, is no better than a placebo.

This outcome alone may not convince everyone that vertebroplasty is a bad thing. Who cares if the effect is "in your head," as long as it works? Some with expertise in the placebo effect would hold this position. Although vertebroplasty was no better than a sham procedure, either may very well be better than doing nothing. In this book we examine other interventions that claim to decrease pain but perform no better than a sham procedure. In many cases, both are better than doing nothing. What does this mean? There is something about the acts of a medical intervention—the thoughtful counsel of the doctor, the skilled support of the nurses and staff, the psychological comfort of acting—that collectively make us feel better. The downside is only that the procedure is costly, may involve risk (either because of the procedure itself or by delaying an intervention that has intrinsic benefit), and involves deception. The question then becomes, Can we reap the benefits of placebo treatments without the deception, the risk, and the cost? In chapter 2 we discuss the placebo effect in more detail. For now, let us at least agree that the money spent on the cement used in vertebroplasty—often thousands of dollars per procedure—was wasted. Salt water would have sufficed.

When medical reversal involves pills or procedures, it affects patients unlucky enough to have an illness and be prescribed a faulty therapy. When reversal involves prevention efforts and screening campaigns, millions of healthy people can be affected. In the past five years, two major public health efforts, breast and prostate cancer screening, have, to a large extent, been overturned. Let's consider mammography.

In 2009 the U.S. Preventive Services Task Force, generally considered the most impartial of the hundreds of groups that produce guidelines for physicians to follow in their clinical practice, changed its recommendation on whether women in their forties should undergo screening mammography. The old recommendation was to do a mammogram in this age group every other year. The new recommendation is not to do it at all.

This reversal made a lot of people very angry. An article from November of that year in the Seattle *Times* had the provocative title "Mammogram Mania: Risking Lives or Dollars? Physicians' Community Speaks Up, against New Recommendations." Radiologists, who had the most to lose (at least financially), protested the loudest. They accused the task force of trying to save money instead of lives.

Was any of this a fair characterization? Were the changes to the guidelines a shock? Not to those who had followed the medical literature. The truth is that the guideline change was three years in the making.

In 2006 a huge study on exactly the question of mammographic screening for 40-somethings was published in *Lancet*. More than 160,000 women in their forties were randomized to mammography screening, or not, and they were followed for, on average, 10.7 years. It is worth pausing to consider just how impressive a feat this study was. The study authors got more than 100,000 women to participate in a study of a medical treatment that required yearly visits for over a decade. For reasons we discuss later, as far as evidence in medicine goes, this is about as good as it gets.

The authors of the trial found that there were fewer deaths from breast cancer among the women who received mammograms, compared to those who did not, but this difference did not reach statistical significance. In other words, the difference was so small that we cannot be sure the difference was not due to chance alone. What this means is that a few women who got mammograms died of breast cancer and a few women who did not get mammograms also died. Neither group had more women who died of breast cancer.

If you look at the study for what is truly important, dying, from any cause, not just breast cancer, you find that the death rate was identical in the two groups. Therefore, we should not screen these women with mammography, because in the history of medicine no one has ever shown that doing so saves lives. In aggregate. On the whole. Regardless of the financial impact.

Put another way, what if all the women in their forties of Washington, D.C., got mammography and all the women in their forties of Chicago did not. Well, nearly all the women in this age group in both cities would be alive at 50, and a few unlucky ones in each city would have died of breast cancer. And all the statisticians at the NIH in Bethesda, Maryland, and at the University of Chicago would be hard-pressed to say for certain which city got mammograms if you did not tell them. If the statisticians looked at death rates for 40-something women in both cities, they would be identical.

What led to all the hand-wringing about the guideline changes was not the reversal of screening mammography; it was that doctors had recommended mammography for women in their forties for all those years. A costly, ambitious medical program was conducted on a national level for years before we had data that said that it worked. What we know for sure is that because of false-positive mammograms and a phenomenon called "overdiagnosis" (more in chapter 4) the program gave many women a cancer scare, a needle biopsy, radiation exposure, surgery, or worse.

We believe that reversal is the most important problem in medicine today. When we doctors flip-flop on our advice to patients, it usually is not because the treatments stopped working. It usually is not because someone discovered a harm no one had previously noticed. It is usually because the practice never worked—we were wrong all along. We promoted it before we had properly studied it. We knew it had some harms, sure, but we never thought it lacked benefits. This problem underlies people's distrust of the medical establishment and is a very important reason that health-care costs are soaring without any improvement in people's health.

Now reversal is not the only problem in medicine, but it is a common channel through which many of the problems run. Yes, pharmaceutical companies manipulate data to get drugs and devices approved and used. Yes, physicians overtest and overtreat for fear of malpractice suits and because of the financial benefits that this behavior brings. Yes, hospitals and clinics market tests and treatments that offer little benefit because they believe they will attract well-insured patients. However, if we find a solution to the problem of medical reversal, a way of preventing the use of therapies that do not work, many of these other problems will cease to exist.

WHAT IS TO COME

In this first part of the book, we describe many reversals and estimate the frequency of medical reversal. We describe the harms of our broken system. Many are obvious, but there are some surprising harms of medical reversal. The repercussions may go further than you imagine. In part 2, we provide you with an understanding of evidence-based medicine, an understanding that will prepare you for the remainder of the book and allow you to question the next report about a "revolutionary new treatment." Part 3 focuses on the causes of medical reversal. Money, of course, is involved, but in this case it is not the entire problem. The seeds of reversal are sown at the start of medical school and are nourished throughout the medical industry.

In part 4 we propose solutions for the problem of medical reversal. Our solutions are not a checklist and a vague call for you to *be prepared* when you see the doctor. We show just where changes can be made to medical education, medical research, and the process by which treatments are approved, so as to eliminate ineffective therapies. We also offer suggestions about how individuals can become better consumers of health care, how to be people who are unlikely to want, or be given, treatments that do not work. Because fundamentalism, in all its forms, is dangerous, we end by discussing those times when it is not necessary to demand that practices be based on ironclad data.

We hope that through reading this book you will understand the scope of the problem of medical reversal—how reversal affects every part of the doctor-patient relationship. This understanding may very well change your opinion of "feeling better." It will certainly affect what you do when you feel well, in order to stay healthy, and what you do when you feel unwell.

2

SUBJECTIVE OUTCOMES

:: WHY FEELING BETTER IS OFTEN MISLEADING

IN CHAPTER 1 WE DISCUSSED FIVE examples of reversal. Four of these—flecainide after heart attacks, stents placed in the coronary arteries of people with stable angina, atenolol as a treatment for hypertension, and mammograms for women in their forties—were similar in that they failed to improve what are considered objective end points. These are end points that we can easily measure: life events (death, heart attacks, or strokes), lab values, or other measurable variables (weight, blood pressure). The fifth reversal we discussed was quite different. Vertebroplasty was intended to improve a subjective end point. It was supposed to help people's pain.

Doctors cringe every time a new study makes headlines announcing that the treatments we have been prescribing do not work. Patients feel even worse, often becoming confused, angry, and skeptical. These reports usually tell us that the treatment does not improve an objective end point: the blood-pressure pill that was supposed to reduce mortality really does not. It confounds everyone even more when a treatment that was meant to improve a subjective end point is reversed. When the study came out reporting that the vertebroplasty procedure did not work, a woman who had the procedure for a spinal compression fracture—an ailment that had been causing a great deal of distress right up until the procedure—might say, "What do they know? Let me tell you, it works." The response of her doctor to these results would be similar. "I don't care what the study says, I do this procedure and I know my patients feel better afterward."

Disbelief is strongest when it comes to medical reversals that have to do with how people feel. When a reversal occurs because a treatment that was supposed to save lives (but had never been shown to) is proved ineffective, we cannot be very surprised. Sure, we thought it made sense mechanistically, but we never really had evidence of efficacy. When a treatment that was supposed to make people feel better, and did seem to make people feel better, is shown not to, that is devastating. Doctors assumed the intervention worked because their patients told them that it did. That seemed like evidence enough. This chapter presents multiple examples of these sorts of reversals.

In the era of evidence-based medicine, medical research has not given subjective end points the importance that they deserve. This is ironic, since most people go to the doctor to feel better. Doctors often pursue treatments that improve survival while making patients miserable in the process. Patients usually have precisely the opposite goals—they value feeling better much more than living longer. So when a new study suggests that the procedure that made you feel better actually had no effect—well, that is a pill that is hard to swallow.

THE CHALLENGE OF JOINT PAIN

As an example of how surprising one of these reversals can be, imagine this. You are 55 and have some knee pain that has been going on for about six months. It started out of the blue, is moderate in severity, and X-rays you had looking for osteoarthritis were pretty normal. With some rest and ibuprofen, your knee feels better, but the need to favor it during your regular activities is beginning to frustrate you. At a follow-up visit, your doctor suggests an MRI (magnetic resonance image) because he thinks your exam is consistent with a meniscal tear. The MRI shows a degenerative tear, one caused not by trauma but by wear on the knee. Your doctor suggests that you have surgery to repair this. He tells you the knee finding is abnormal, that it is easily repaired with a "relatively noninvasive surgery," and that you will be better after the procedure. Hearing this, you eagerly agree. After an outpatient surgery followed by a home exercise regimen, you are feeling better. You think, "Boy, that was the right thing to do."

Before discussing why this procedure, arthroscopic knee surgery to repair degenerative meniscal tears, is a wonderful example of a therapy that does not work—despite having been done for years to improve a subjective end point—let's consider some background. The menisci are small pieces of cartilage, nicely described as crescents, that sit inside our knees. They allow the joint to move smoothly and disperse the forces that the knee must bear every time we take a step. The menisci sometimes tear. Tears can be traumatic (you have almost certainly heard of athletes missing whole seasons after meniscal tears) or degenerative. Degenerative tears are much more common. These tears sometimes occur as our knees age, and they are becoming increasingly common as our society grows older and heavier. Arthroscopic surgery is a minimally invasive orthopedic procedure in which the surgeon operates through scopes placed inside the joint through small incisions.

Arthroscopic surgery to repair degenerative tears of the menisci is big business. Each year in America, 700,000 patients undergo the procedure with the goal of relieving pain. The price tag for all these procedures is $4 billion a year. You would think that a procedure this common must work.

However, in 2013 two studies specifically examined arthroscopic knee surgery. The first found that surgery followed by physical therapy (as is always done) was no better than physical therapy alone. The study suggested that starting with a noninvasive approach would markedly decrease the need for surgery. The results of the second study was even more striking. This study found that surgery was no better than sham surgery. The researchers randomly assigned patients with degenerative meniscal tears and no osteoarthritis to sham surgery or to actual surgery. Patients randomized to the sham procedure went to the operating room. While there, the surgeon inserted the scopes, looked around in the knee, and generally pretended to do surgery. A patient who had sham surgery was in the operating room for the same amount of time as one who had real surgery. Both groups went on to have physical therapy. There were no differences in pain and functioning at 2, 6, or 12 months after the procedure.

So if arthroscopic surgery to repair degenerative meniscal tears does not work, why have patients and doctors sworn by it? When it comes to feeling better, we have known for years that procedures can elicit a placebo effect. What is the placebo effect? A placebo is any intervention that is not known to have, or intended to have, physiological benefits. A placebo might be a pharmacologically inert sugar pill or an ineffective intervention such as a sham surgery. When patients are given a placebo and have an improvement in their condition, beyond what is expected with a tincture of time, we call that the placebo effect.

The placebo effect is real and has been supported in many studies. There have even been successful efforts to determine the underlying physiology of the effect. In a famous study in the 1970s, patients undergoing surgery for impacted molars received placebos for postoperative pain. When the patients whose pain responded to the placebo were given the drug naloxone, a drug that blocks the effect of morphine, the benefit of the placebo disappeared. This study, along with similar ones, strongly suggests that the placebo response is due to real physiological changes in the body. When we are experiencing pain, our brains secrete endorphins, which are natural substances similar to morphine. The placebo effect is, however, not universal. Attempts to define an average placebo effect, by analyzing the effect in many, varied studies, have been unable to determine one. That said, it does seem that the placebo effect is most common when it comes to therapies meant to reduce pain and that the effect tends to be relatively short-lived.

Because the placebo effect is strongest for subjective end points (nobody has ever proved that a placebo can make you live longer), we must make sure that studies of treatments meant to improve subjective end points are perfectly controlled. The participants in the control arm of a study (those people not getting the treatment) need to receive an intervention that is as close as possible to the real thing, so that both the treatment group and the placebo group attain an equivalent placebo effect. For instance, comparing surgery to exercise would not be a good study. After recovering from the surgery, you may feel better even if the surgery did not help. You will feel better because you expected to, you wanted to, and you were told by someone you trusted that you would. The appropriate study is comparing surgery to the most comparable thing—sham surgery.

THE ROLE OF SHAM SURGERY

If arthroscopic surgery to repair degenerative meniscal tears does not work, even though it seemed like it did, what about other orthopedic procedures? Consider those procedures that are so common we do not even imagine that they may not work? The anterior cruciate ligament (ACL) is one of the four ligaments that hold the knee together. It is commonly torn in sports (football, soccer, skiing) and is generally repaired without a second thought. We fix it because it is broken and because it seems to make people better. It has, however, never been rigorously tested—meaning it has never been tested in a randomized controlled trial with a sham-surgery arm. It turns out that the vast majority of orthopedic procedures for pain still have no sham-controlled studies. As a specialty, orthopedics has been reluctant to perform rigorous studies with sham-surgery controls.

Often the ethics of sham surgery is used as justification not to do these studies. Is it ethical to perform a sham procedure? Consider the converse question: is it ethical not to do a study with a sham-surgery control? When we institute a practice without this sort of evidence base, as we did with the meniscal surgery discussed earlier, we perform an operation half a million times a year, collecting billions of dollars, without any idea whether it even works. Estimating even a minimal complication rate of 0.1 percent for arthroscopic surgery (infection is an inevitable risk with any surgery), at least 500 people each year are suffering from a procedure that does not work.

Although it might seem extreme to question procedures that reasonably ought to work (and appear to work), the evidence supports skepticism. Reconstruction of torn ACLs might be the next procedure to be reversed, or at least to become less common. A study in 2010 randomized young, healthy people with recent ACL tears to early ACL repair with physical therapy (the current standard of care) or physical therapy followed by ACL repair only for those patients who did not get better. It turned out that with this approach, about half of the patients were able to avoid surgery. It will be interesting to see the results of the obvious follow-up study: patients with ACL tears all receive physical therapy, and those who do not get better are then randomized to ACL repair versus sham repair. The results might surprise us.*

SUBJECTIVE END POINTS OTHER THAN PAIN

Studies of vertebroplasty and arthroscopic surgery to repair degenerative meniscal tears demonstrate the power of sham procedures in untangling the complicated way our bodies experience pain. But what about

---

* If you wonder why we are taking physical therapy for granted, you are catching on. Is physical therapy really better than just telling patients to exercise at home? Or maybe, do nothing at all? Seems like something worth testing, too.

other subjective end points? Is pain unique in its susceptibility to place-bo response? Let us consider one of the most common ailments to affect healthy people: asthma. Nearly 300 million people worldwide carry a diagnosis of asthma. The treatment of asthma is a mainstay of any internist's or pediatrician's practice. During the throes of an asthma exacerbation, people become acutely aware of their breathing; they suffer with wheezing, chest tightness, and shortness of breath. People with asthma are quick to recognize the power of two puffs of the potent medicine albuterol. Delivered as an aerosol, albuterol dilates the airways, relieving the symptoms of asthma.

A study in the *New England Journal of Medicine* comparing asthma treatments is instructive when we consider treatments aimed at improving subjective end points—in this case shortness of breath. People in this study were randomized to four different therapies: an albuterol inhaler; a placebo inhaler; sham acupuncture; and no intervention. After use of the treatment, both objective and subjective end points were evaluated: spirometry, a test of how well air moves out of the lungs; and a questionnaire asking patients how they felt. The objective measure of lung function was no surprise: only albuterol improved how much air patients could move. The subjective outcome results, however, were a bit of a shock. Patients reported that all three therapies were better than doing nothing and all three were equally effective.

What this study shows is that even when considering how good you think your breathing is, the placebo response is robust. Those of us without lung problems rarely even know we are breathing. However, for people with asthma, breathing can take center stage. Asthmatics can often tell you whether their breathing is normal or "a little tight." Even among these people, who are highly attuned to their own bodies, the placebo response can rival an active drug. This study encourages further caution toward interventions that claim to make us feel better.

The take-home lesson is that we have to be skeptical of even the practices that make us feel better. We need to test these interventions to make sure the effect is real—an effect of the treatment itself, not just the effect of being told that the treatment works. You might argue, "If people feel better, who cares if the response is a placebo response." That argument is reasonable. In fact, every doctor-patient interaction benefits from the placebo effect. When we, as physicians, see patients and prescribe effective medications, our patients also benefit from the belief that the medications will help them. It is unlikely that a doctor has ever given you a medication and said, "This pill has been shown to work, but I doubt it will do anything for you." This is not just true of practitioners of traditional, Western medicine; practitioners of complementary medicine may rely on the placebo effect to an even greater extent.

AN ACCEPTABLE PLACEBO?

There has been quite a bit of ethical debate over the years about using placebos. We think a few things limit their use as an acceptable medical practice. First, people see doctors to receive proven therapies, not treatments that might work. Going back to the days of patent medicines and snake oil is not something many of us would favor. Second, there may be real harm associated with prescribing treatments whose only effect is that of a placebo. If placebo interventions are expensive, potentially harmful, or delay or replace proven therapies, their use is clearly unethical. In today's world, especially in the world of American health care, it is hard to imagine a placebo therapy, prescribed by a doctor, that is not expensive, does not carry some risk of harm, or does not replace a more effective, proven therapy.

Ted Kaptchuk, a professor at Harvard, is an expert in the placebo effect and has spent much of his career studying its nuances. One of his recent studies aims to convince even the most ardent skeptic how the placebo effect might be used appropriately. As we mentioned in chapter 1, one of the major quandaries regarding placebo therapies has to do with the use of deception. Deception seems integral to achieving the placebo effect, and a modern cornerstone of medical ethics is that deceiving patients is never acceptable. Few of us wish to return to the days when doctors would fail to tell patients their cancer was terminal, or even that they had cancer.

Kaptchuk sought to test whether the placebo effect would still work even without deception. He decided to select an ailment about which there is widespread belief that psychological stressors played a role. He chose irritable bowel syndrome, or IBS.

IBS has a worldwide prevalence of 10 to 15 percent and is one of the top 10 reasons people go to the doctor. It is a gastrointestinal disorder characterized by abdominal discomfort, and, depending on the person, constipation or diarrhea or both. Little is known about the biological cause of the disease, but for years the observation was made that the placebo effect can lead to improvement in the condition. For this reason, Kaptchuk selected IBS as his laboratory.

In a study, 80 people with IBS were randomized to two groups. Half received no treatment, and the other half received a sugar pill and were told that the pill had "self-healing properties." All other treatments for IBS (such as laxatives or antidiarrheal medications) were continued. Remarkably, people who received a sugar pill and were told that this was a pill made only of sugar had a statistically significant improvement in their IBS symptoms and felt better than those who did not. Kaptchuk proved that even without deception, the placebo effect could occur. As he put it, "Our results challenge 'the conventional wisdom' that placebo effects require 'intentional ignorance.'"

What does this study tell us? A couple things. First, no one believes a placebo is acceptable if it is extremely costly (vertebroplasty, orthopedic surgery), delays proven therapies, or causes real harms. We can debate whether or not deception is permitted in select medical circumstances, and one might argue that if a placebo is cheap, proved to be better than the alternative (doing nothing), and patients are fully informed of what they are getting into (no deception), then, under those circumstances, placebo treatments can be considered. While vertebroplasty was unacceptable, what about sugar pills for patients with IBS?—this is less clear. Our bias is toward abandoning them, but we also believe there is no single right answer and much room for debate. There may be a role for promoting a low-cost placebo in a setting of total transparency.

THE SUBJECTIVE NATURE OF ANGINAL CHEST PAIN

Now, let's apply these lessons to a final example using a truly classic medical experiment from the 1950s that tested a costly and invasive medical practice. Consider angina, which in chapter 1 plagued Anthony Baker. Anthony's cardiologist placed a stent to open up a clogged artery—which everyone agreed was the source of the problem. Anthony felt better after the procedure and was happy to have a new lease on life. He left the office thinking that the stent would improve his survival (studies show that many patients believe this). Then, as we indicated, it was proved that stenting these lesions did not help patients live a single day longer. The study was named COURAGE.

When Anthony heard this news, he was disappointed. Well, he reasoned, at least my pain is better. In fact, a follow-up publication from the COURAGE study shows just this. Placing stents in the coronary arteries of people with stable angina reduces chest pain and improves quality of life, somewhat, at 6, 12, and 18 months. By three years the benefit of the treatment wanes, and the study shows that pain is identical between the people who had gotten stents and those who were treated only with medicine. Fine, Anthony says, even if the benefit is small and short-lived, at least there is some benefit to the procedure. All in all, he is happy to have had it done. Many doctors agree with this reasoning. They fault the medical system for throwing the baby out with the bathwater. Even if stents do not make you live longer, you live better, they argue. That counts.

Without a doubt, that counts. If placing stents in the coronary arteries reduces chest pain, people should have that option as a way of treating their pain (as long as they realize that is the only benefit). However, the problem with COURAGE data for chest pain is that, in studying this subjective end point, the control arm was inadequate. The COURAGE trial tested whether stents improved pain compared to medications. But getting a stent is a major intervention. A cardiologist talks you through the procedure and then you are sedated. Often, you are shown your angiograms afterward. You see an image of a clogged, disfigured artery transformed into an open pipe with beautiful flow. How could such a convincing improvement in the plumbing not improve symptoms? To truly see whether stenting improves pain, the control arm should be a sham coronary-artery intervention. Patients randomized to the control arm should have everything except the stent placement. In arthroscopic knee surgery and vertebroplasty, that was what it took to reveal the placebo effect. You might be reluctant to do this study. Angina is different from knee pain, you might argue. It has to do with blood flow. There cannot be a placebo response in angina, can there?

Consider a study from 1959. In the years leading up to this seminal *New England Journal of Medicine* paper, doctors struggled with angina. They knew it was a problem with blood flow in the coronary arteries, but they did not have the tools or the medicines to really address the problem. One proposal was that if you tied off (ligated) the internal mammary artery, an artery in the chest that does not lead to the heart, there would be increased upstream flow to the coronaries. It was a bold idea that was not without a physiological basis.

In 1955 an Italian team tried the procedure, internal mammary artery ligation, on 11 people with severe chest pain. The results were impressive; all 11 had improvement in their pain. By 1959 the same team of doctors had treated more than 300 people. Most were doing well.

Then in 1959, Leonard Cobb published the results of his classic study.
He had recruited patients with angina and brought them to the operating
room to perform the procedure. At the point in the surgery when it was
time to ligate the artery, the researchers randomized the patients to ligation
or sham ligation. Those patients who had sham ligation were told the procedure had been done when it had not. Of the people who had the ligation
procedure, 32 percent improved; 43 percent of the patients who received
sham operations also improved. A similar study was later published confirming these results, and internal artery ligation was abandoned.

In retrospect, the lesson of Cobb's study was not that ligation of the
artery did not work but that any subjective end point, knee pain in osteoarthritis, shortness of breath in asthma, and yes, even angina in people with
coronary-artery disease, is remarkably susceptible to the placebo response.
If the patient believes the treatment will work, often it does work.

With this in mind, we can look at the results of the COURAGE trial with
a bit more skepticism. The benefit in symptoms was small and completely
lost by 36 months. The control arm received medicine alone, not a sham
procedure, the closest thing to the procedure. Could stenting for people
with angina from stable coronary-artery disease be like ligation of the internal mammary artery? Could the small, relatively short-lived benefit simply
be a placebo effect? There is no answer to that question, not without a definitive study, but we can say the idea is plausible enough to consider. It should
be tested. If stenting were found to be no better than sham stenting, then
percutaneous coronary intervention for people with stable angina would be
the greatest example of reversal, at least in terms of cost, in the past 20 years.

CONCLUSION

Reversals of treatments that made us feel better are disconcerting. We put
tremendous faith in knowing how we feel, and it is confusing to find out
that our own bodies can fool us (and our physicians). All the practices that
we discussed really did make people feel better. However, in each example
it was not really the treatment that helped; it was the idea of the treatment.
This would not be a problem if our placebo therapies were cheap, carried
no risks, did not involve deception, and had no potential of delaying receipt
of therapies that would be more beneficial. Therapies that were thought
to benefit objective outcomes can be overturned; likewise, therapies that
affect subjective outcomes can be reversed.

3 SURROGATE OUTCOMES

THOMAS GALBRAITH WAS DISAPPOINTED. He had just gotten off the phone with his endocrinologist and his numbers were still too high. The doctor told him that a measure of his average blood sugar, the hemoglobin A1c (HbA1c), remained "above goal."* It sounded ridiculous to Thomas. He had been doing everything right: eating well, watching his weight, and taking all his diabetes medications, which now totaled three pills and one shot of insulin each day. Thomas was a 64-year-old accountant who had, as we say in the business, multiple medical problems. He was overweight, had diabetes and high blood pressure, and had experienced a heart attack a few years earlier. Now, he also had an HbA1c of 7.5 percent—"above goal." His doctor wanted the number below 7.0 percent. Thomas's doctor told him that he would need to increase his insulin dose and emphasized that a lower blood-sugar level would improve his chances of avoiding another

---

* The HbA1c measures the percentage of hemoglobin, a normal component of our blood that has sugar attached to it. In people with normal levels of blood sugar, 3 to 6 percent of the hemoglobin is "glycated." When the blood sugar is elevated, as in diabetes, this percentage goes up.

heart attack (as well as many other sordid complications that the doctor seemed to enjoy enumerating).

That night over dinner—steamed green beans and baked tilapia—Thomas discussed the situation with his wife. Despite losing three pounds over the past three months, not missing a single pill (which now included pioglitazone, saxagliptin, and metformin), and taking his five units of insulin at bedtime, his HbA1c was a percentage point above where his doctor wanted it to be. He recounted what his doctor had said—for every 1 percent rise in HbA1c, his risk of stroke or heart attack went up nearly 20 percent and his risk of death went up 12 percent.

This whole scenario was playing out in May 2008. Thomas redoubled his efforts to lose weight. He grudgingly increased his insulin (which seemed to make him feel a bit foggy in the morning) and dedicated himself to an even more ascetic diet. After all this, it came as a shock when in June of that year Thomas read about a study. This study concluded that the lower HbA1c his doctor wanted would not *reduce* his risk of death; it would actually increase it. And his HbA1c of 7.5 percent was better for him in the long run than anything below 7.0 percent. "Are you kidding me?" Thomas asked, as he read the news story.

THE TRUTH ABOUT SURROGACY

In the first two chapters we presented reversals that involved objective end points, like heart attacks and death, and subjective ones, like knee pain and back pain. Now we are discussing another sort of end point—the surrogate end point. Surrogate end points are a whole different matter. Many of the reversals that we have discussed, and will discuss, occur because we have adopted therapies whose efficacy is supported by inadequate data. Surrogate end points are at the heart of a generous portion of that inadequate data.

Strictly speaking, surrogate end points are objective ones. They are end points that we can easily and directly measure. Surrogate end points, however, unlike clinically important objective end points, are invisible to the patient. They are stand-ins. We use them because it is simpler to show that a treatment improves a surrogate end point than to show it improves a real clinical one. For this reason, the medical literature is full of surrogate end points. It is easier to show that a drug improves bone density than it is to show that it decreases the rate of fractures. It is easier, and far less expensive, to show that a drug lowers blood pressure than it is to show that it decreases the rate of strokes. It is easier to show that a drug lowers blood sugar than it is to show that it decreases the risk of blindness, kidney failure, heart attacks, and death. Studies with surrogate end points may require dozens of patients and take months to years; studies with clinical end points often require hundreds of patients and need to run for years or even decades.

Thomas's story illustrates what can happen when we rely on surrogate end points. What went wrong in this case is that HbA1c is not a perfect surrogate for what we are really interested in: all the harms that diabetes can do. Thomas is really not interested in lowering his HbA1c, and with an HbA1c of 7.5 percent he is not having any symptoms of diabetes. What he is interested in is lowering his risk of diabetic complications, such as going blind or dying of a heart attack. We have already presented a couple of reversals that were linked to the use of surrogate end points in chapter 1: antiarrhythmic drugs decrease the number of premature ventricular contractions but do not improve survival after a heart attack, and atenolol lowers blood pressure but does not improve survival.

The surrogate end points that appear in the medical literature are varied: many are measurements made in the lab (cholesterol levels and HbA1c); others are measured by procedures: electrocardiograms (premature ventricular contractions), blood-pressure measurements, or CT scans (tumor size). In what follows, we provide a tour of surrogate end points to demonstrate just how common and how tricky they can be.

Returning now to Thomas. After he read about this study in the news, he began to wonder why we adopted HbA1c as a surrogate marker in the first place? Turns out that doctors used the best observational studies of people in the real world and paired that information with their biological understanding. They first asked a simple question: Which patients with diabetes do best? When you ask that question, it turns out that people with HbA1c readings less than 7 percent live longer (and better) than those with higher levels. The researchers realized that this made perfect biologic sense; the closer the average blood sugar was to that of a normal person, the less damage the blood sugar would do to the organs. After this relationship was seen in countless studies, doctors began to recommend an HbA1c of less than 7 percent as the goal for most people. Some doctors strove for even lower numbers.

Doctors were so convinced of the benefit of a low HbA1c that they codified it into law—or the closest thing to law in medical practice—clinical guidelines. Many medical practices used the HbA1c as a measure of how well doctors were managing their patients with diabetes. *Hey Doc, bad news, only 28 percent of your diabetic patients have an HbA1c below 7.0 percent. Do you think you can do better?*

When we discuss the types of studies that we base decisions on in medicine (in chapter 9), we consider why observational studies, such as the ones that defined the association between low HbA1c and better outcomes, can be problematic. However, you may already begin to see why this is true. A person in the "real world" with a lower HbA1c might do better not because of the lower numbers, but because she is the sort of person who does better. In other words, if you have a strong social network, are wealthy, live in a good neighborhood, have a personal trainer, and generally are healthier, your HbA1c might be lower naturally. It might very well be everything else in your life (everything other than the low HbA1c) that makes you better off. Of course, these issues can get very confusing. If you have all these advantages, you might also have access to better health care, which would put you in touch with doctors who believe that a lower HbA1c is better. These doctors might be pushing you toward a lower HbA1c with medications. This might actually be harming you. But, because of all the other advantages in your life, you still come out ahead. As we said, it can get very confusing.

HbA1c seemed to be an especially robust, well-validated surrogate marker because it was not just observational studies that predicted its utility. A few randomized trials, real experiments, demonstrated that bringing people with diabetes to HbA1c values of 7 to 7.5 percent was better than leaving their HbA1c's at 9.0 percent or so. Of course, these were different populations of people (some even had type 1 diabetes, really a very different disease from Thomas's type 2 diabetes), who were sometimes treated with different drugs.

The study that got Thomas's blood boiling was the ACCORD trial, published in 2008. ACCORD was a randomized study in which doctors enrolled more than 10,000 people with diabetes and divided them into two groups. Half had their sugar lowered to a goal of below 8.0 percent, basically the standard of care, and the other half aimed for an HbA1c below 7.0 percent. The standard-of-care group achieved an average HbA1c of 7.5 percent, while the intensive-treatment group achieved an HbA1c of 6.5

percent. As expected, the group with a lower sugar target, the "intensive" therapy group, used more drugs to achieve their goal. They often ended up on medical regimens similar to Thomas's. At the end of the study, there was no difference between the groups in terms of the combined rate of death from a cardiovascular cause, heart attacks and strokes. There was one difference in outcomes between the groups: there was a clear difference between the two groups in terms of overall mortality. In one group, 4 percent of the patients died; in the other, 5 percent died. Unexpectedly, the group with a higher death rate was the intensive-treatment group.

The findings of ACCORD were bolstered by a similar study called ADVANCE, which found that patients achieving a goal HbA1c of 6.5 percent did not live longer than those achieving an average HbA1c of 7.3 percent. Targeting a goal of less than 8.0 is no worse (and possibly better), when it comes to survival, than targeting a goal of less than 7.0. Thomas's doctor, although with good intentions, was telling him to do the wrong thing.

HOW TO TREAT CHOLESTEROL

Studies in every corner of medicine rely on surrogate markers, and no discussion of the topic would be adequate without talking about hypercholesterolemia, or high cholesterol. This surrogate marker has essentially become accepted as a disease in the United States. You do not feel your cholesterol level. You may feel terrible after a fatty meal—we all do—but it is not cholesterol you are feeling. Cholesterol is an important molecule: it makes up part of your cell membranes and the backbone of key hormones. There are different cholesterol molecules. For decades we have known that people with low HDL cholesterol and high LDL cholesterol do worse than patients with the opposite combination. When we say worse, we really mean worse. They have more heart attacks, more strokes, and a higher death rate. This relationship is so clear that we commonly refer to HDL as good cholesterol and LDL as bad cholesterol. Much of the information about cholesterol comes from the Framingham Heart Study, a famous study in which a large group of men and women (mostly white) from Framingham, Massachusetts, were studied for more than 40 years.

Given the close relationship between people's cholesterol profile and their health, it was not much of a leap to assume that lowering cholesterol would improve health. Many drugs have been developed to achieve this goal. Among the most commonly used drugs in the United States are the statins, a class of drug that lowers cholesterol and, most definitively in patients with high cholesterol and heart disease, saves lives. The success of statins is especially satisfying because earlier medications, some tested in the 1980s, seemed to improve cholesterol numbers without improving people's overall health.

This last fact suggests that cholesterol level might not be a perfect surrogate for cardiovascular disease. This has been borne out recently. Extended-release niacin was approved in 1997 based on its ability to raise good cholesterol (HDL), and lower bad cholesterol (LDL). Fenofibrate received Food and Drug Administration (FDA) approval in 2001 based on data showing that it could lower bad cholesterol (LDL). Despite the success of both of these drugs in improving people's cholesterol levels, neither has proved to actually help people.

In 2010 fenofibrate was tested in a trial of more than 5,000 people with type 2 diabetes. All these people were given a statin medication and then randomized to fenofibrate or a placebo pill. This was a beautiful study because it mimics precisely how doctors use this medication in the real world—to lower the cholesterol levels of an at-risk patient who is already on a statin. After 4.7 years, 2.4 percent of patients in the placebo group had had a heart attack, stroke, or death related to the cardiovascular system. In the fenofibrate group, 2.2 percent of the people experienced one of these outcomes. These probabilities were statistically indistinguishable. Fenofibrate improved cholesterol levels but failed to improve the end points we care about most; the drug improved a surrogate end point but not an objective, clinical one.

Similar data regarding extended-release niacin were published a year later. In this trial, more than 3,000 patients with persistently low good cholesterol (HDL) were randomized to niacin or placebo. As in the previous trial, all patients were also given a statin. At two years, niacin had raised good cholesterol by seven points but did not improve the study's primary end point, a smorgasbord of bad things, "death from coronary heart disease, nonfatal myocardial infarction, ischemic stroke, hospitalization for an acute coronary syndrome, or symptom-driven coronary or cerebral revascularization." In 2014 yet another study cast doubt on niacin.

If these two studies looked only at surrogate end points, like so many earlier studies did, they would have concluded that these drugs impact cholesterol favorably and therefore both should work to reduce heart attacks and strokes. But because these trials went further, and asked directly whether the medications improved clinical end points, they were able to give us true, albeit disappointing, answers. The lesson when it comes to cholesterol is the same as the HbA1c lesson—improving the numbers is just that, improving numbers. It does not necessarily translate into what we care about, helping people live longer or better.

We should add that the examples we have highlighted do not show that niacin and fenofibrate do not work under *any* circumstances. They just show that they do not work in the circumstances under which they were tested. These circumstances mirrored how the drugs are used in the real world, and it is under these circumstances that proponents assert the drugs should work. Like millions of other chemical compounds in the world, these medications may improve some outcomes under some conditions (in some patients, with a certain array of risk factors), but as of 2015, just how they can help remains to be seen. And, as should be true for all medicines, until a treatment is proven to work, there is no reason to assume it does and use it blindly.

The problem of surrogate end points goes beyond blood tests like HbA1c and cholesterol. In chapter 1 we saw how a common medication, atenolol, successfully lowered blood pressure, a surrogate outcome, but did not reduce deaths.* Two more examples extend the argument to an even more diverse set of surrogates. The first is progression-free survival in the treatment of cancer.

BEVACIZUMAB IN BREAST CANCER

Metastatic breast cancer is a terrible disease. It is a cancer that, either because of its biology or its time of detection, has spread beyond the breast to other organs of the body. That is what we mean by metastatic. We treat metastatic breast cancer with chemotherapy drugs that slow the growth of the cancer cells. The goal is not to cure the disease—at this stage that is impossible—but to control it and allow patients to live longer. In the

---

* Blood pressure is an interesting example. It is a surrogate because we usually cannot feel it and it is used as a stand-in for a host of dreadful cardiovascular outcomes. At extremely high levels, though, blood pressure can cause symptoms and thus becomes an objective, clinical end point.

very early 2000s, a new drug called bevacizumab (Avastin) was added to the menu of chemotherapy options for metastatic breast cancer. Bevacizumab is actually not a chemotherapy drug but a monoclonal antibody that changes the way the blood vessels inside cancer grow.* Some experts believe bevacizumab can decrease blood-vessel growth inside tumors, thus robbing them of the nutrients and oxygen that they need to grow. Others believe that the drug may work by improving the delivery of chemotherapy to the cancer. Regardless of the precise mechanism of action, it has become one of the most studied and used drugs in cancer medicine.

Patients and doctors came to believe that bevacizumab, when added to more traditional chemotherapy, could help women with metastatic breast cancer. In 2008 the U.S. FDA granted bevacizumab accelerated approval for this purpose, based on evidence that it improved progression-free survival in breast cancer.

What is progression-free survival? Progression-free survival, or PFS in oncologists' lingo, is an end point that means the patient has survived and that her cancer has not progressed. Progression is defined as growth of a tumor by more than 20 percent of its initial size as measured by a CT scan. If the patient is alive and the tumor has grown by 19 percent or shrunk by 16 percent, that outcome counts as progression-free survival. In studies, the survival portion of the end point is typically of lesser importance, as it usually makes up just a fraction of the total PFS: of all the people who either progress or die, most have progressed, but only a few have died.

PFS is a surrogate end point. Do patients feel progression? Not really. Often patients feel bad as their cancer returns, but no one can tell you, "OK, I have crossed the arbitrary 120 percent threshold and now I have progressed." Sometimes patients feel bad at 101 percent, and sometimes they feel fine up to 160 percent.

Does PFS predict improved overall survival—a longer life span? If it did, it would be a very good surrogate end point. Turns out, the answer to this question is complicated. A British group called the National Institutes for Clinical Excellence commissioned an analysis of this question. The analysis looked at all the studies that compare PFS to actual survival. There

---

* Monoclonal antibodies are proteins that bind to a specific target. Antibodies are naturally produced by our immune system to bind to foreign substances like bacteria. They can also be produced in the lab to deliver drugs to a specific substrate, such as cancer cells.

was huge variability among the studies—depending on which study you picked, PFS and actual survival either correlated very well or not at all. The outcome of the National Institutes for Clinical Excellence's analysis: "We need more research." But for the specific question of metastatic breast cancer, the answer is clearer. The correlation between PFS and survival is poor in nearly all published analyses.

In the case of bevacizumab, the value of PFS as an end point was critical. The U.S. FDA approved bevacizumab in breast cancer based largely on a trial showing that, when added to chemotherapy, bevacizumab improved PFS. It improved it a lot, nearly doubling PFS, from 5.9 to 11.8 months. In this particular cancer, that is a sizable improvement. What was unexpected in this study was that survival barely changed. It was around 26.7 months for those who received bevacizumab and 25.2 months for those who did not. But at the time, since the PFS benefit was so large, many doctors assumed that meant we would eventually see a true survival benefit or, at a minimum, a benefit in terms of quality of life. The drug became widely used.

Just three years later, however, the FDA reversed its decision, voting against bevacizumab's use in metastatic breast cancer. After looking at two more trials, the FDA found that bevacizumab may increase PFS but not actual survival. Tumors hit the 20 percent growth mark later, but patients did not live a day longer. The women who took this drug suffered side effects, had better CT scans (for a while), and ultimately did not benefit. No matter whether PFS and overall survival correlate well *on average*, bevacizumab taught us that PFS is still a surrogate that can be misleading.

Surrogate end points generally have two qualities. First, they are well correlated (or we think they are well correlated) with a clinical end point. We know that people with lower blood sugar, better cholesterol profiles, and slower cancer progression do better than those with higher blood sugar, worse cholesterol, and more rapidly progressive cancers. Second they make perfect biological sense. Of course, bringing blood sugars close to normal will improve outcomes in diabetes, especially since we know that it is the high sugars that do damage. It is also these two facts that make it so surprising when surrogates turn out not to be predictive—when they improve with an intervention but the real, clinical end points do not. A final example of a misleading surrogate end point is one that was especially surprising because it made such perfect sense: improving blood flow in people who have suffered a heart attack.

BLOOD FLOW AS A SURROGATE MARKER

Some heart attacks are mild. They cause only brief discomfort, injure a small portion of the heart, and leave its function nearly intact. Other heart attacks are massive, leaving the heart unable to pump normally. This life-threatening situation is called cardiogenic shock. The patient has dangerously low blood pressure and a very high risk of death. Doctors take cardiogenic shock very seriously. We use medicines and intravenous fluids to improve blood pressure, we do everything we can to open the blocked artery that caused the heart attack, and, often, we place an intra-aortic balloon pump (IABP).

The IABP was invented in the 1960s and was truly ingenious. The IABP is a long balloon that is inserted in the aorta, the large artery into which the heart pumps all of its blood. The balloon is connected to a computer that controls when the balloon inflates and deflates. The balloon inflates when the heart is filling with blood and deflates when it is pumping. IABPs are clever because both their inflation and their deflation assist the heart's function. When the heart pumps into the aorta, the balloon deflates rapidly, creating a vacuum and drawing the blood forward into the peripheral circulation—toward the rest of the body where the oxygenated blood is needed. The deflating balloon acts like someone sucking on a straw, in this case, the aorta. When the heart is not pumping, the part of its cycle when it fills and rests, the balloon inflates. This not only pushes blood forward into peripheral circulation, but it also pushes some blood back to the heart, potentially giving this same oxygen-rich blood to the arteries that supply the heart muscle itself. Early studies supported this theoretical physiological benefit.

Over the years, the IABP steadily gained popularity. The idea was that because it helped a surrogate outcome, cardiac output—the volume of blood being pumped by the heart—it would help patients with a low cardiac output. Recent international guidelines (recommendations for doctors) said that placing an IABP should be part of the care of patients with a heart attack and cardiogenic shock. Because of this, as of 2010, up to half the patients who fit this description had an IABP placed. You know where this story is going, don't you.

In 2012 the IABP SHOCK II trial enrolled 600 patients with cardiogenic shock caused by a heart attack. All the patients received the best care available. Half also got an IABP. The results were surprising. At 30 days, 40 percent of the patients had died (this is a very serious condition) and the pump made no difference at all. Not only did IABPs not save lives, they also did not improve any of the end points the researchers examined. They did not reduce the rate of second heart attacks in the hospital, or stroke, or complications of the procedures to open the blocked artery that caused the first heart attack. The IABP is another example of a therapy, adopted because it made really good sense and improved a surrogate outcome, that failed to improve the end points that really matter. It is also worth noting that the IABP is a costly intervention that can have significant complications (as you might expect if you imagine inflating and deflating a balloon in the aorta).

There are some interesting points about IABPs. First, we include IABPs in our discussion of surrogate markers because the procedure improved cardiac output, a stand-in for a real clinical end point, preventing death.* Second, the IABP is an intervention instituted not only because it improved a surrogate end point but because it *seemed* like it should work. The mechanism of the treatment was just so darn elegant. We discuss this phenomenon in great detail later when we examine the causes of reversal. Lastly, there was also some hint that doctors were suspicious of the effectiveness of IABPs. Although guidelines supported their use, only 25 to 40 percent of patients with cardiogenic shock actually received them. Make no mistake, that is a lot of balloons, but for some reason 60 to 75 percent of doctors were not following this guideline.

HOSPITALIZATION IS, AMONG OTHER THINGS, A SURROGATE

We end this discussion with a final type of surrogate end point, one that is both a surrogate and an end point of importance in and of itself. A small group of unfortunate people in America are frequently hospitalized. These people often have conditions that get better and worse, such as heart failure or emphysema. When things are going well, these conditions can be managed at home. But when things are going poorly, these are common reasons for admission to the hospital. Since patients are hospitalized because

---

* The improved cardiac output was noted in early studies of the device, although more recent studies suggest that the pump might not even improve the surrogate.

they are doing poorly, many doctors believe that the end point that matters most for these people is a decrease in hospitalization.

Hospitalization is tricky. All things being equal, it is better to avoid being hospitalized. Anybody who has spent any time as a patient in a hospital knows that it is not where you want to be. Putting aside that you usually feel terrible while you are hospitalized, there are the issues of the food, the noise, and those gowns—not to mention the risk of infection, medication errors, and potential adverse effects of all of our 21st-century interventions. So, in part, avoiding hospitalization is an objective end point. However, many doctors read more into it. They argue that it is also a surrogate end point. The fewer times you are hospitalized, the less likely you are to die. Used this way, hospitalization is a surrogate for death.

Lars Hemkens and colleagues wanted to test the second part of this statement. Of course, all things being equal, it is better not to be hospitalized. But is it possible that some intervention could decrease the rate of hospitalization while paradoxically increasing the death rate? This was the puzzle they set out to solve: was hospitalization also a good surrogate for death?

To do so, the group studied both hospitalization and death across a large collection of trials where both were reported. They found that one-third of the time, when hospitalizations went down, mortality went up, or vice versa, meaning that a treatment that prevented hospitalization made you more likely to die; something that seemed like a bad intervention (after all, it increased hospitalization) actually made you live longer. This analysis is thought-provoking because few people would have even considered hospitalization to be a surrogate marker. But, of course, in part, it is. Findings like this allow doctors to give more nuanced guidance to patients as they choose what they consider to be the most important outcomes. Their conclusion was that mortality and hospitalization are both important and both should be reported in studies. It is a mistake to assume that one implies the other. In this sense, hospitalization—like so many other measurements we have looked at—is not a reliable surrogate end point for the most important outcome: living longer.

CONCLUSION

Surrogate end points come in many forms, some obvious (HbA1c, hypercholesterolemia) and some less so (hypertension, hospitalization). They are attractive because they are relatively easy and inexpensive to study.

They also usually make intuitive sense. But sometimes, maybe often, they do not correlate with the outcome that we care about.

Throughout this book, we make the case against surrogate end points. We argue that the way to prevent reversal is to have good evidence that medical practices improve hard end points—the ones that we care about. It is entirely possible that we will someday have perfectly reliable surrogate end points, but that achievement will involve a great deal of hard work. To prove that a surrogate is perfectly reliable will require many studies of hard end points, demonstrating that the surrogate always gets it right. We have yet to see such assurance for any surrogate end point, and recent history has given us ample reason to be skeptical for the time being.

4
SCREENING TESTS

AFTER USING THE BATHROOM, Christopher D'Amico carefully folded a square of clean toilet paper and tucked it in his underwear. This was routine—just a precaution—a perennial reminder that he was not a young man anymore. Ever since his prostate cancer treatment, Christopher had struggled with a little incontinence. It was not too bad, nothing a little toilet paper couldn't handle, and, all in all, it was a small price to pay to be alive.

Three years earlier, at age 63, Christopher had gone to see a urologist. For months before this visit, he had been waking two or three times a night to use the bathroom. From the drug ads on TV, he knew these were probably symptoms of benign prostatic hyperplasia, BPH. BPH occurs in up to half of middle-aged men. Among other things, this enlargement of the prostate can cause incomplete bladder emptying and nighttime trips to the bathroom. Christopher did not have a regular doctor, and a friend suggested that he go straight to a specialist.

The urologist took Christopher's history, examined his prostate, and, as expected, diagnosed him with BPH. Before Christopher left the office, the doctor drew blood to screen him for prostate cancer. A few days later Christopher got a call telling him that his prostate specific antigen (PSA) was elevated, meaning that in addition to BPH, he might also have prostate cancer. A week later, Christopher was having biopsies of the prostate. A few days after that, the urologist called to say it was cancer.

Cancer. The big C. Just hearing the word gave Christopher shivers. His father, an inveterate drinker, had died from esophageal cancer. His older brother, a longtime smoker, had lost his battle with oral cancer the previous year. And, now, he thought, it's my turn. His children were still in college; he was still working to support them, and his wife needed him. I've got to beat this, he said to himself.

A few weeks later, Christopher underwent surgery. The surgeon was a robot. Well, not exactly—his surgeon was actually a nice guy, but he controlled a robot during the surgery. The robot did the actual cutting.*

Christopher recovered well from the surgery, and his PSA went to zero—the prostate cancer was cured. The only lingering effects were the incontinence and impotence. Although he still desired sex, Christopher really could not get any sort of useful erection. This was an unfortunate side effect, but Christopher's doctor told him his life was saved because the cancer was caught early. It all seemed worth it.

A few years later, Christopher began to have mixed feelings about the surgery and the PSA blood test that led to it. Some of his friends told him that they had had long conversations with their doctors about the risks and benefits of prostate cancer screening and ultimately decided to forgo the PSA test. Christopher asked, "Didn't the test save lives?" Well, it wasn't so clear, his friends told him. Then Christopher read in the newspaper that a major task force had announced that before routinely performing the PSA test, doctors and patients should have a conversation about it. A few years later, Christopher turned on the radio to hear that the same group of experts now advised men not to get a PSA at all. Each time he tucked the toilet paper into his pants, Christopher was reminded of how little he understood about that blood test, which had either saved his life or made it worse.

In the first three chapters, we have explored major categories of medical reversal. For practices meant to make us live longer, we have seen rever-

---

* Many advertisements attest to the benefits of futuristic-sounding robotic surgery, but at least for prostate cancer, there is no good evidence that patients do better if a robot helps their surgeon.

sal happen when evidence supporting a practice was weak or flawed. This included times when the evidence relied on surrogate end points. For practices meant to make us feel better, we have seen how powerful the placebo effect is and noted reversals when treatments were later tested using appropriate controls, such as sham procedures. Screening recommendations have also been reversed. In many ways, reversals that involve screening are the worst kind. Unlike medical therapies, screening tests are performed on healthy people. An ineffective screening test will affect not only a few people with a disease who are seeking treatment, but an enormous number of healthy people who just want to stay that way. An ineffective screening test can turn millions of healthy people into patients.

Screening for a disease just seems to make sense. We suggest screening tests because they offer the promise of prevention. We have been brought up on the proverb "An ounce of prevention is worth a pound of cure." It is hard to accept that such a simple and sensible mantra might not apply. When it becomes clear that it does not, screening tests become the subject of real controversy. The controversy is magnified because screening guidelines do tend to change. Even the most evidence-based screening guidelines, often made by the U.S. Preventive Services Task Force (USPSTF), will almost certainly be modified in the years to come for legitimate reasons as new data become available. Understanding screening—what it is, why we do it, how we know when it is beneficial, and the controversies that surround it—requires understanding three related topics. The first is the most basic: the goals of screening and the evidence that supports some of our most commonly done tests. The second is overdiagnosis, a counterintuitive phenomenon that often undermines our best efforts. The third is how screening tests perform in the real world, outside of the studies meant to support or refute their utility.

GOALS AND EVIDENCE FOR SCREENING

What is screening, and why do we do it? Screening for a disease means going out and trying to find a disease early, before it has caused symptoms. We screen large numbers of healthy patients to try to find a disease. The logic is that if we find a disease early, detect a cancer when it is small, we can cure it. We screen for diseases only because we hope that if we find and treat them early, people will live longer than if we waited until the disease became symptomatic to treat it.

The history of screening, specifically cancer screening, goes back more than 100 years. In the early 20th century, when surgery was the only way to treat cancers, surgeons realized that patients diagnosed with large tumors usually died, while those with smaller ones sometimes lived.* The earliest cancer-education campaigns, therefore, sought to teach people how to recognize cancer at its earliest stage. This was the beginning of cancer screening. As time went on, evidence suggested that we could do even better. Though diagnosing a small tumor is good, diagnosing a cancer before it has become a cancer is even better. The hunt for "precancerous" or "premalignant" lesions is the basis of Pap smears and modern colon cancer screening. In our current age, we have gone from screening for the anatomic (visible lesions) to the microscopic (precancerous cells) to the molecular (abnormal genes). Today there are debates about whether we should treat people who have abnormal genes—who are at risk for cancer—with procedures like prophylactic mastectomy.

We now have recommendations to screen for diseases as diverse as diabetes, hepatitis C, coronary-artery disease, and HIV. Cancer screening, however, is what is advised most broadly in practice and is what people talk about most. For that reason, we focus on it. The principles we discuss apply to all screening interventions. Cancer-screening tests, such as mammography (breast cancer), the PSA blood test (prostate cancer), colonoscopy (colon cancer), CT-scan screening (lung cancer), and Pap smears (cervical cancer) are designed to catch cancer when it is treatable. Colon and cervical cancer screening aim to detect premalignant lesions, while breast, prostate, and lung cancer screening really try to detect small, curable cancers. Doctors believe that, left alone, these precancerous lesions or early cancers would grow larger and spread, eventually killing you—taking many years of the life you otherwise would live. An effective cancer-screening test should thus accomplish three goals:

1. It should find cancers early.
2. It should lower the rate of dying from the cancer it is meant to find.
3. It should improve overall survival (decrease the rate of dying from anything).

* Ilana Löwy's book *Preventive Strikes: Women, Precancer, and Prophylactic Surgery* (2010) provides a wonderful description of how screening got to where it is today.

A screening intervention cannot accomplish goal 2 unless it can accomplish goal 1. It also cannot accomplish goal 3 unless it accomplishes goal 2. Goal 3 is what really matters. People are screened for cancer—have mammograms and colonoscopies—only to live longer. Goals 1 and 2 are only means to an end, steps toward an ultimate goal. Imagine if a test effectively finds a cancer, decreases the rates of death from that cancer, but doubles or triples the rate of heart attacks. If, on the whole, people die sooner, it does not matter how effective that test is as a cancer screen.

How do we test screening tests? Ideally, screening tests would be tested with randomized controlled trials. We have mentioned these trials already, and we discuss them in quite a bit of detail in chapter 8. In a trial of a screening test, tens of thousands of people would be divided into two groups. One group would get the screening test and the other would be simply monitored. We would then follow the groups to see if the screened group lived longer than the group who was not screened—goal 3 from the list above. At this time, when it comes to screening tests, we usually do not have that kind of data. For some tests the trials just have not been done; for others, the results of studies do not show us what we expect. Obviously, practicing without this sort of evidence base means that we may be recommending things that do not actually work. We leave ourselves open to the possibility of future reversal.

Any screening test that you have heard about accomplishes goal 1: it finds cancers early. Colonoscopies, PSA testing, mammograms, Pap smears, and now CT scans for lung cancer find cancers before they become detectable by the patient or that patient's doctor. Surprisingly, the evidence showing that common screening tests accomplish goal 3 (and even goal 2) is pretty weak. To begin with prostate cancer, some randomized trials (but not others) have shown that PSA testing reduces dying from prostate cancer (goal 2) but have not shown that it makes people live longer (goal 3). This was partially behind the USPSTF's decision to stop recommending PSA testing.

Randomized trials of mammography have shown that this screening test reduces the chance of dying from breast cancer (goal 2). These findings, however, are quite variable, with some trials reporting large reductions and others reporting only small ones. Mammograms probably do not decrease the risk of dying of breast cancer for women in their forties. Whole books have been written about the mammogram question, but suffice it to say that mammography has not been shown to improve overall survival (goal 3) at any age.* As it stands, the USPSTF only recommends mammograms every other year for women between ages 50 and 74.

Pap smears have for years been the standard to which screening tests are compared. This test has likely saved innumerable lives around the world. Because this test came into use before the advent of evidence-based medicine, it has not been rigorously tested in randomized trials. One trial we do have studied a one-time Pap smear in rural India. Although this trial did not show a benefit in terms of death rates related to cervical cancer (goal 2), a one-time Pap smear is not what doctors do in the United States, so it is hard to apply this study to the developed world. Even without good data, the idea that Pap smears save lives is widely held, but there is a lot of debate regarding how often they need to be done—once every three years, every five years?

If you are over 50, your doctor has almost certainly recommended a colonoscopy for colon cancer screening. Colonoscopies are currently being tested in randomized trials, and the results should be back in the early 2020s. Two other ways to screen for colorectal cancer have been tested, and the results from these trials have been extrapolated to colonoscopy. Sigmoidoscopy and fecal occult blood testing (a way to look for microscopic drops of blood in the stool) have both been shown to reduce the risk of dying of colon cancer (goal 2) but not the risk of death overall (goal 3). The USPSTF presently recommends colon cancer screening for people from age 50 to 75.

The new kid on the block is CT-scan screening for lung cancer. This test is a little different from the others we have discussed, because instead of being offered to everybody over a certain age, it is recommended only for a group at high risk, specifically people between the ages of 55 and 80 with a heavy-smoking history. This test has been shown to reduce overall death rates as well as death rates from lung cancer (goals 3 and 2, respectively). This is the only screening test to date that makes you live longer. Even here there are some caveats. Most of the abnormalities that are found with this test, and thus demand evaluation, turn out to not be cancers. (In one study, 96 percent of abnormal findings were false alarms.) Also there is the intriguing finding that the total number of lives saved by lung cancer

---

* A terrific book on the subject of breast cancer screening is *Mammography Screening: Truth, Lies and Controversy*, by Peter Gøtzsche (Radcliffe, 2012).

screening seems to be greater than the lives saved from treating lung cancer. In other words, the improvement in goal 3 was bigger than the improvement in goal 2. How a screening test for lung cancer saves lives beyond its effect on lung cancer needs to be understood. This is an odd result.

Putting aside CT-scan screening for lung cancer, which applies only to a relatively small group of people, why have no other trials of screening tests shown improvement in all causes of mortality? There are two possibilities. The first is that these trials are not powerful enough to see a difference. For instance, in studies of colorectal cancer with 30 years of follow-up, for every 10,000 people, 192 people die of colon cancer in the unscreened arm, while 128 die in the screened arm. This is a statistically significant difference that shows the beneficial effect of screening. However, when you look at overall mortality, not just mortality related to colon cancer, 7,109 out of 10,000 die in the unscreened group versus 7,111 out of 10,000 in the screened group. This is not a significant difference. Seeing a statistical difference in the overall mortality is harder and may require many more participants in the trial. This explanation is what most experts believe is happening. It is a reasonable argument and certainly one potential explanation.

The other possibility is that the gains in preventing deaths from cancer are offset by deaths from other causes. Maybe screening for prostate cancer decreases prostate cancer deaths but increases deaths from heart attacks. To understand how this might happen, we must turn to the second concept of cancer screening: overdiagnosis.

OVERDIAGNOSIS

Most experts agree that all cancer screening leads to some amount of overdiagnosis. Overdiagnosis occurs when some of the cancers that are found through screening are insignificant. They are cancers that have no potential to make people sick or die. If a person had not had a screening test, these cancers would have gone undetected and he would have been no worse off. Over time he would have felt nothing and would have died of something else. To Americans, who seem to have a fear of cancer and the need to fight it at all costs written into our DNA, this might seem shocking. That said, there is no doubt that overdiagnosis is a reality.

A simple case might be the best way to illustrate the concept of overdiagnosis. Consider a person who is screened for prostate cancer. He is terribly unlucky: the screening test finds a cancer; he is treated for it; and then he dies of a heart attack the following year. Had this man not been screened for prostate cancer, he still would have died of a heart attack a year later and that cancer would never have caused problems.* Sometimes the cancers we find with screening are so small and grow so slowly that 1 year becomes 20 or 30 years, and dying from a heart attack becomes dying from heart attack, or pneumonia, or a car accident, or even a different cancer altogether. In other words, if you find really slow-growing cancers with a screening test, there is a good chance they are not destined to affect a patient's life expectancy. For all people with these cancers, the treatment for the cancer provides no benefit. They would have lived just as long, dying on the same day they otherwise would have, of something else entirely.

Can we tell which cancers are the overdiagnosed ones and which are the deadly ones? We hope that someday we will be able to, but currently there is no way to distinguish one from the other. Because of this, all screening programs find a mix of deadly cancers and "sit and do nothing" cancers. The ratio of these cancers is of critical importance. In prostate cancer, the ratio tends toward the "sit and do nothing" cancers. When we screen for prostate cancer, we end up treating around 40 cancers for every cancer that will kill.† For mammography, the ratio between dangerous and harmless cancers is contentious. The best studies suggest that if a mammogram finds breast cancer, and it is treated, there is a 13 percent chance that the mammogram will have saved a life. This means that for every one dangerous cancer diagnosed and treated there are eight harmless ones. Most of the cancers we find, when screening for breast and prostate cancer, would have gone unnoticed if not for screening.

Why is overdiagnosis problematic? Overdiagnosis is expensive and potentially dangerous. Presently, we spend almost $8 billion a year on mammography screening in the United States. A large part of that goes to finding cancers that we did not need to find. Cancer treatment is not benign. It often involves radiation, surgery, and hormonal therapy. If screening is finding many unimportant cancers, people are being exposed to this treatment unnecessarily. The side effects of these treatments worsen their qual-

---

* Most would argue that he was worse off having been screened. By having the screening test, he lived his final year of life as a cancer patient.
† This number also takes into account the fact that treatments are not universally effective.

ity of life. Thirty to forty men with prostate cancer experience side effects of treatment in order to lengthen one life. Some side effects shorten lives. If the side effects reduce life spans (by just a little bit), we might break even—saving lives from the cancer while taking a life with the treatment.

You may think this is all a theoretical and unsubstantiated worry. Unfortunately, there is evidence that screening for prostate cancer *does* increase the rate of death from non–prostate cancer causes, specifically from cardiovascular death and suicide. This sort of reasoning, balancing quality and quantity of life, is part of why the USPSTF recently changed its recommendation for prostate cancer screening, now recommending that men do not get screened. For mammography screening, many experts think the testing is favorable if you are 50 to 69 years old but probably not if you are in your forties. For the same reason, the USPSTF advised against routine screening in the younger age group. This was a controversial decision in 2009, but it has been supported by recent data.

POPULATION DATA

The final important topic to understand about screening is population data. This means moving away from the experimental trials and looking at data from the real world. For our discussion, we will focus on breast cancer and prostate cancer because these been evaluated most rigorously.

Population data have undermined our faith in the effectiveness of our screening tests for these two cancers. There are two numbers that really tell the story: the incidence of early cancers and the incidence of advanced cancers. Incidence is the number of *new* cancers that are diagnosed in a given year—how many people were told, for the first time, they have cancer. Early cancers are those that are contained within the breast or prostate. Advanced cancers are those that are found after they have spread from the organ of origin. These are metastatic cancers and are generally very bad. If you find advanced cancer, the thinking goes, you found this cancer too late. If screening works, we should find more early, localized cancers and fewer advanced cancers.

Because the population is always growing, incidence is always reported as a number out of 100,000 people. That way if the size of the United States grows from 200 million to 300 million, the incidence of prostate cancer over time can be compared, for instance 171 per 100,000 in 1990, and 145 per 100,000 in 2010.

Whenever you debut a screening test, you expect the following. Immediately after the test begins to be used, the incidence of early cancer should rise, as you detect cases of cancer that otherwise would have gone unnoticed. This is the definition of screening. Next, after several years, as screening gets adopted throughout the population, the incidence of early cancer should peak and then drift back to nearly the baseline incidence—the incidence prior to the introduction of the test. Figure 4.1 shows this graphically. We say that we end at nearly the baseline incidence because, over time, we are still catching the same number of total cancers as we did before, but some of the cancers we are catching early rather than late, when they are advanced cancers.

For advanced cancer, you expect the following. Immediately after a test is debuted, the incidence of advanced cancer goes up. This is because when you begin screening, you catch some cancers that have already spread. Then, over the next 10 or 20 years, the beneficial effect of screening sets in. In a few decades, the incidence of advanced cancer falls because you are now finding cancers early, curing these patients so they no longer end up with a new cancer that has already spread. Some 20 years after a screening test is put into practice, the patients missing from the advanced-cancer totals should be in the early-cancer figure. (This is the "nearly" from the paragraph above.) Figure 4.1 also shows this.

When it comes to breast and prostate cancer, the curves have not followed this nice pattern. Instead, they look much more like the light gray curves in figure 4.2. Incidence of early cancer did rise after the PSA test and mammography were debuted, but they did not return nearly to baseline. They stayed well above the baseline. This would be a good thing if all of those extra cancers that were found translated into a marked decrease in advanced cancers. In fact the rates of advanced cancer have fallen, but only by a very small amount. Putting this together, it means that we are finding *many more* early cancers than the advanced cancers we are preventing. This means we have overdiagnosis. The surplus of early cancer represents people who would never have known they had cancer had it not been for the test. These people experience all the downsides of a cancer diagnosis—surgery, radiation, chemotherapy, anxiety—with none of the benefits—a longer, healthier life.

The actual graph for breast cancer is shown in figure 4.3. In the years before mammography, for every 100,000 women, doctors diagnosed 112 early cancers and 102 advanced cancers each year. After 30 years of mam-

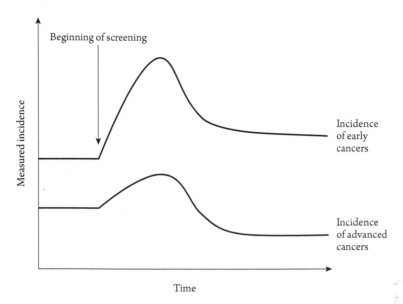

4.1 How a screening test should work.

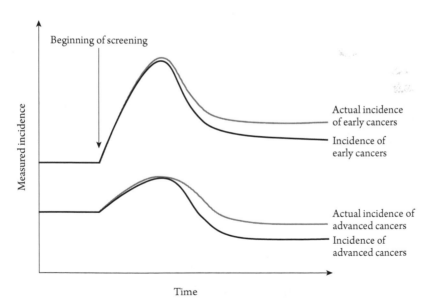

4.2 What actually happened with breast and prostate cancer screening.

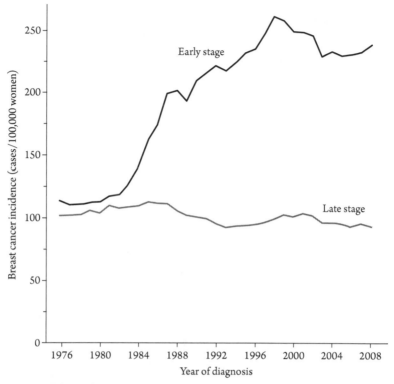

4.3 Actual data on breast cancer since mammograms became commonly used.
Source: Bleyer A, Welch HG. Effect of three decades of screening mammography on breast-cancer incidence. N Engl J Med. 2012;367:1998–2005. Copyright © 2012, Massachusetts Medical Society. Used with permission from the Massachusetts Medical Society.

mography, we find 234 early cancers each year. The rate of diagnosis of advanced cancer has declined to 94 per 100,000. So each year, 122 extra cases of early breast cancer are found (234 – 112 = 122), for a reduction of 8 cases of advanced cancer (102 – 94 = 8).

In the real world, by screening for breast and prostate cancer, we have found many more early cancers, with a disappointing impact on advanced cancers.

REVERSALS IN SCREENING

Taking these factors into consideration, we can return to medical reversal. Only CT-scan screening for lung cancer currently reaches the highest standard of proof that a cancer-screening test is beneficial—that it actually saves lives (which does not sound like such a high standard). Mammography for women in their forties was once universally recommended, but USPSTF withdrew this recommendation in 2009. This test is still commonly done. Prostate cancer screening was once widely recommended and used. This recommendation was first narrowed to younger age groups before being withdrawn altogether.

These reversals occurred slowly, not with a single study but as advisory groups concluded that the risks and benefits, which once seemed favorable, now seem less so. Seminal trials paved the way for these changes. A 2006 study published in *Lancet* found that mammograms did not improve breast cancer mortality among women in their forties in the United Kingdom. A study from Canada published in 2013, covering a wider age group, showed similar results. And these studies dealt with *breast cancer mortality*, not the more important overall mortality. Recent trials in prostate cancer have followed a similar trajectory.

The definitive way to settle the question of the effectiveness of screening tests is to conduct clinical trials large enough to see whether screening for cancer improves overall survival—not breast cancer survival or prostate cancer survival. Such trials would likely require over a million participants. Because such so-called megatrials may be costly, many people think they are improbable. However, the history of medicine has shown us that studies that are important do get done in the long run, despite the challenges. And a better way to think about the price tag for the megatrial is to remember that each year in America, we spend hundreds of billions of dollars on screening tests and their downstream costs. Spending a small percentage of this money to show whether these screening tests are actually helping people is a small price to pay.

THE FUTURE OF SCREENING AND HOW WE, THE SCREENED, SHOULD PROCEED

Over the next decade, we think it is very likely that we will see a continued pullback on recommended screening tests. The benefit of mammograms, for those at average risk for breast cancer, will probably be shown to be negligible. Guidelines for cervical cancer screening will continue in their present direction, recommending more and more time between tests. Medicine's experience with breast and prostate cancer screening means that future screening tests will have to meet an appropriately high bar before being adopted. We would like to see a time when a test needs to show that it saves actual lives before it is instituted.

In chapter 17, we discuss how to protect yourself from medical interventions that are likely to be reversed. In terms of screening tests, people should never be screened in ways that are more aggressive than the USPSTF recommends. Even for the recommended screening tests, it is important that we have informed conversations with our doctors. People should understand how likely a screening test is to help them personally, what are the potential harms—both physical and emotional—of the test, and, most importantly, what the test has actually been proved to achieve.

5
SYSTEMS FAILURE

BY NOW, WE HOPE you are becoming suspicious of unproven medical interventions. Many treatments that seem like they should work do not. It does not matter whether the treatment is a pill, a procedure, or a screening test—many seemingly reasonable and accepted interventions have failed. Before moving on from the ineffective therapies in which doctors have placed their faith (and on which they have staked their patients' health), let's consider one more category: systems interventions. One family's experience serves as an example of a systems intervention that failed.

THE PEOPLE INSIDE THE SYSTEMS

Joanne Murphy often thinks about her husband. It has only been a year since Carl died from leukemia. He was a 30-year veteran of the local police force, a youth soccer coach, a man who could fix anything, and a fine and loving father. When Carl first fell ill, his daughter was in her final year of college. One of his greatest concerns was that his illness would disrupt her studies.

As expected, the illness and the therapy were difficult. Although the doctors and nurses were incredibly kind to both Carl and Joanne, being in the hospital for weeks on end for treatment was exhausting. Carl tolerated the lousy mattress, the 4:00 a.m. blood draws, and the incessant beeping of machines. He endured painful mouth sores, rashes, and episodes of fever. He even accepted the food and the pathetic scrap of fabric they called a blanket. One thing that did bother Carl, mainly because he could never make sense of it, was that he was placed on contact precautions for vanco-mycin-resistant enterococcus (VRE).

VRE is a really nasty bacteria, one that is resistant to many antibiotics. As standard practice, during one of his admissions, a nurse swabbed Carl's skin. That swab revealed that Carl was colonized by VRE. It was not making him sick, just living on him, as countless bacteria do on all of us. Just how and when Carl got this bug, no one could say, nor did it really matter. What did matter was that now the doctors and nurses had to stop at the door to Carl's hospital room, open a cart, take out a yellow paper gown, put it on over their clothes, and then put on gloves before entering. This was not to protect Carl, but to protect other patients by halting the spread of this dangerous species of bacteria.

The list of things about this "glove and gown protocol" that irritated Carl was long. First of all, although the whole process was brief, lasting only about a minute, he could tell that it frustrated everybody. Once the members of his health-care team were in his room, he noticed that people's behavior was inconsistent. Some people were very careful about "covering up," while others would sit on his bed, allowing their uncovered pants to touch his sheets. Occasionally, people would forget the gown altogether—sometimes these people would just pop in to fiddle with a beeping intravenous pump or collect a breakfast tray, but other times they would sit and talk.

Beyond the inconsistency, the gowns and gloves bothered Carl because he was suspicious that they meant that fewer doctors visited his room. One junior physician, a friendly young lady, had been in the habit of coming by to sit and talk before she went home. After the VRE test, she would only stand at the door and say hello. Both of them understood that she wanted to visit but could not stay long, and it probably was not worth the whole ordeal of dressing up.

On one occasion Carl asked a doctor how much those yellow dresses cost. The doctor said a few dollars each. That cannot be right, Carl thought; it is basically a giant yellow paper towel.

Joanne and her daughter actually found Carl's list of irritations charming. He had always been unfailingly friendly and chatty, as well as a real stickler for details. He was also known to be . . . thrifty. The things that annoyed him about the gowns were the things his wife and daughter loved about him.

One night, surfing the web, Carl found an article about a study that confirmed his suspicion. Doctors were less likely to visit patients on "contact isolation." It made perfect sense. Who wants to bother with all that? Carl was actually sort of satisfied to have been proved right, and he figured, "Well, if helps keep other patients safe, I can tolerate it."

Carl died from his leukemia a little less than a year after he was diagnosed. Subsequently, two articles were published that would have angered him. In 2011 researchers found that similar gown-and-glove precautions did not decrease the transmission of VRE or methicillin-resistant Staphylococcus aureus (MRSA, another dangerous bacteria) in intensive care units (ICUs). This was a study of more than 3,000 patients in 19 ICUs who received universal screening for these bacteria (the same type of screening that identified Carl's VRE). The second study (an impressive entry into the acronym arms race: the Benefits of Universal Glove and Gown, or BUGG study) found that making all health-care workers wear gowns and gloves also did not reduce transmission of VRE or a combination of VRE and MRSA (the study's goal).* In short, both studies suggested that all this "gowning and gloving" does not really help decrease the spread of dangerous bacteria. Carl put up with an intervention he did not like, that made him feel a bit like a pariah, which may have led to fewer visits and potentially worse care and likely did not benefit other patients.

WHAT ARE SYSTEMS INTERVENTIONS?

This type of reversal affects something relatively new in medicine: the systems intervention.[†] More and more these days, we recognize that good medical care requires more than just a good doctor. It takes a skilled team

---

* There was a small difference in the rate of acquisition of MRSA, but this finding was less convincing, since it could have been that the ICUs assigned to "gown and glove protocol" had much higher rates of MRSA before the study began. It was also not the study's primary end point.

† Systems interventions in medicine go by many different names: systems innovations, quality interventions, and health-delivery interventions.

of doctors, nurses, and affiliated health-care professionals to deliver today's often complex care. Conversely, when things go wrong, it is usually not that a single individual fell short but that the system was designed poorly and an error either was not caught or was actually magnified by other people's actions. Systems interventions stem from this evolution in health care. We think that we can overcome many flaws in health care if we improve the systems of health-care delivery. Gown-and-glove precautions are an example of a systems intervention. Other examples include checklists for surgical teams, procedural rules, quality measures, public reporting of outcomes, and economic incentives. A systems intervention is a change in how health care is delivered, one that affects how groups of caregivers act or behave in their professional role.

Businesses use systems interventions all the time. They use them to improve workplace productivity, to improve the quality of products, and to produce products at lower costs. Businesses recognize that these interventions are made in the real and messy world of human beings and thus lend themselves to unintended consequences. Sometimes they do not have the desired effect; sometimes they have the opposite effect. What looked good on paper may not work when instituted in the supply chain or on the factory floor. Businesses therefore continually reevaluate their interventions, willing to abandon what does not work—the interventions that generate cost but no benefit.

In contrast to the business world, systems interventions in health care are often adopted without a real plan to study them. They make good intuitive sense and are often backed by indefatigable proponents. After "successful" adoption, these interventions may even come to be mandated at a national level. Given the unusual way that health care is paid for in the United States, these interventions exist in a world not governed by traditional market pressures. Once adopted, therefore, they can be very difficult to modify.

All this would be fine if systems interventions always achieved their desired goals (even with a few unintended consequences). But as was the case with the gown-and-glove intervention, these interventions are frequently shown to be ineffective. They become examples of medical reversal. The problem is compounded because even a well-done study showing ineffectiveness tends not to be the end of a systems intervention. There are often vocal proponents who are not dissuaded and argue that the intervention would have worked if only you did it a little differently or studied it a little differently. In chapter 16 we will see why this argument (the "it would have worked if only . . ." argument) is flawed, why you must show that something actually works *before* it is adopted. For now, let us consider lessons from other reversals of systems interventions.

WHEN SYSTEMS INTERVENTIONS
BECOME MEDICAL REVERSALS

Multidrug-resistant bacteria are a major problem in nearly every hospital. VRE, MRSA, and similar bacteria can infect vulnerable patients, leading to life-threatening infections or even death. Although gown-and-glove precautions for patients colonized with VRE probably do not work to decrease this problem, medicine should do everything possible to minimize the harm of multidrug-resistant bacteria. We should devise strategies to reduce infection and death from these bacteria. The strategies would probably need to include ones that reduce the overly generous use of broad-spectrum antibiotics. Any promising strategy should be tested in a randomized trial to confirm that it does what is claimed. We err when we implement practices based on a good theory, on the experience of only a few hospitals, or on studies that are not well done—as happened with gown-and-glove precautions. (Despite the studies we mentioned, national guidelines still advise that hospitals employ gown-and-glove precautions.)

Gown-and-glove precautions were adopted largely on the basis of what doctors call *single-center, before-and-after* studies. Single-center means that the study was performed at a single hospital. The proof from such a study tends to be tenuous because a single center may be idiosyncratic. It may have a unique demographic of patients, or bacteria, or an unusually enthusiastic proponent who manages to change the culture in ways that are not reproduced at other hospitals. (Gowning and gloving may actually work, but only when instituted flawlessly.) There have been some major discrepancies between single-center and multiple-center (multicenter) trials. Later in this chapter we discuss one famous one, regarding the control of blood sugar in intensive care units.

Before-and-after studies are problematic too, and they are the initial data behind most systems interventions. "Before-and-after" means that we measure the outcome we are interested in first before and then after we implement our intervention. You may ask, for instance: does the rate of infections associated with intravenous (IV) catheter insertion decrease after we implement a checklist of best practices that includes steps like washing hands, sterilizing the patients' skin, and donning full sterile gowns? (This was precisely the question in a recent before-and-after study.) You measure the rate of infection in your hospital before you institute the checklist and then afterward. The problem with this design is twofold. First, your intervention is never the only thing that has changed in your hospital, so it is hard to separate the effect of the intervention from other trends. The other challenge is something called the Hawthorne effect.

The Hawthorne effect is a psychological principle stating that people perform differently (usually better) when they know they are being watched. This effect was named by Henry A. Landsberger, who studied a series of systems initiatives meant to improve productivity at the Hawthorne Works, a factory in Cicero, Illinois, in the 1920s and 1930s. The most famous initiatives involved altering the level of illumination on the factory floor. Analysis suggested that although the actual interventions at the Hawthorne Works had little or no effect, the simple act of studying people did. Brightening the light on the factory floor helped productivity during the study, but the improvement declined after the study ended, even though the brightness remained.

When doctors and nurses know you are counting IV catheter infections, they start taking their own prevention measures more seriously; they become more vigilant about keeping intravenous sites and tubes sterile. This is a good thing, but a before-and-after study would conclude that the checklist is leading to the improvement when, in reality, the improvement is just a consequence of keeping count of IV catheter infections. The worry with the Hawthorne effect is what happens when the study ends. You might continue to implement your intervention, with all the associated costs (and potential harms) but none of the benefits. Your workers might go back to their baseline productivity, only on a brighter factory floor.

It is worth pointing out that for this particular example, a checklist for safe placement of IV catheters, the decrease in IV catheter infections was dramatic, and subsequent studies showed the benefit was maintained. While these results are welcome, they do not mean that it was the checklist that led to the reduction in infections. The only way to prove that the checklist was the cause would be to randomize hospitals to use the checklist or to simply receive the education regarding how to place and maintain central lines. Let both groups of hospitals know that we are concerned about the rate of IV catheter infection rates and will be monitoring those rates. Then follow the rates of infection over time. In 2012 a report of such a randomized trial was published. After randomizing hospitals to the checklist or routine care, the authors found that both groups achieved a median of 0 central line infections per 1,000 days at the end of the randomized study period. The mean number of line infections was different, as the authors repeatedly highlight in the paper, and that number favored the checklist, but it is hard to know that this is not due to just a few, stubborn bad-apple hospitals in the control group. In short, we have yet to see a very large, well-done randomized trial confirming that it is truly the checklist that makes the difference.

Returning to gown-and-glove precautions, it is clear that these precautions should work. If the problem is that resistant bugs are being spread by clinging to doctors' and nurses' clothing, wearing a disposable cover should help. In before-and-after, single-center studies, gowns did decrease the rate of transmission. And yet, when the policy was tested in a randomized fashion, it did not work. The problem with systems interventions is twofold. First, when they do not work, we spend precious time, energy, and money to keep them going anyway. Second, the intervention adopted without evidence potentially distracts us from truly promising alternatives. In the gown-and-glove case, a different approach may actually decrease the spread of these bugs. Others have tested in a randomized trial whether the use of decontamination wipes decreases transmission of these resistant bugs, and it appears to work. It also appears to decrease hospital-acquired bloodstream infections. There are still questions, of course, but this strategy has already cleared a hurdle (the randomized trial) that gown-and-glove precautions avoided for years, before studies proved the technique ineffective.

Another example of a costly, widely implemented, but ultimately contradicted systems intervention is the rapid-response team, or RRT. Every day, in hospitals around the world, alerts go off that there has been a cardiac arrest. Unexpectedly, a patient who had been doing all right, in a standard hospital room, is now near death. In retrospect, when we look at the patient's vital data in the hours leading up to the cardiac arrest, it often appears that we could have seen it coming. The person's heart rate may have begun to climb hours before; her blood pressure may have dropped transiently two hours earlier; or her temperature might have been rising. You might assume that if we had only acted sooner, we could have prevented the cardiac arrest.

This belief led to the implementation of the RRT. The RRT is usually a group of well-trained nurses, occasionally in collaboration with physicians, who monitor vital signs remotely or are at the ready if called on by a patient's primary doctors and nurses. The hope is that this team will identify patients who are heading for trouble, or they can be called on when the primary team first becomes concerned. The RRT then swoops into a patient's room, makes an assessment, and intervenes before things get worse. The hope, of course, is that the presence of this team will decrease the number of cardiac arrests and improve survival.

The history of the RRT is similar to that of the gown-and-glove intervention. First, a serious problem was noted—in this case, too many seemingly preventable cardiac arrests. Second, a perfectly sensible intervention was suggested, the RRT. Third, single-center, before-and-after studies demonstrated that the RRT decreases cardiac arrests and improves survival. Soon, nearly every hospital in America had an RRT and it was considered a mark of quality.

Then in 2005, the MERIT trial was conducted at 23 hospitals in Australia. The investigators randomized hospitals to either adopt the RRT model or not. They found that although the RRT was well utilized, the number of cardiac arrests, unplanned ICU admissions, and unplanned deaths did not change. Interestingly, both groups had a reduction in cardiac arrests over time. The MERIT trial demonstrated both that RRTs do not work and that we are getting better at treating these patients. The MERIT trial also proved that a systems intervention could be an example of medical reversal.

NEITHER PROVED NOR DISPROVED, THE GRAY ZONE OF SYSTEMS

Gown-and-glove precautions and the RRT are systems interventions that became widely accepted, and good evidence now shows that they do not work.* Certainly, there have been systems interventions within health care that have improved patient outcomes. One recent example is an intervention that instituted careful discharge planning and home visits for a popu-

---

* In neither of these cases, however, has there been a rapid retreat from use of the intervention.

lation of elderly patients leaving the hospital. This intervention decreased multiple outcomes, including rehospitalization. Besides interventions being proved effective or proved ineffective, a third outcome might be most common: the systems intervention is adopted but is neither really proved nor contradicted. The intervention is adopted based on weak data, it persists in practice for years, being increasingly questioned, but it is never conclusively rejected. Over time, equally weak evidence accumulates that the intervention is not achieving its intended goal or is having unintended consequences that outweigh its benefits. These are not medical reversals in the strongest sense, but they are examples of probably ineffective practices being continued for years, until they fall out of favor. There are two informative examples of this sort of practice.

Ten to fifteen years ago, observational studies suggested that among people who go to the emergency room with pneumonia, those who receive antibiotics within four to eight hours have better outcomes than those who receive antibiotics later. In an ideal world, the logical reaction to these data would be to design a randomized controlled trial. You would compare one group of hospitals, where doctors were incentivized to treat appropriate patients with antibiotics as soon as possible, with another group of hospitals that would provide the current standard of care. Your outcomes would include measures of success in treating pneumonia (mortality, length of stay in the hospital) as well as potential adverse effects of the intervention. We do not live in this ideal world, of course. Instead, what actually happened was that without real evidence, the four-hour goal was widely implemented, became a national quality measure, and served as the basis for pilot programs that paid hospitals more based on how well they met this mark. Soon after, people began to recognize unintended consequences. Patients who did not have pneumonia were given antibiotics, and doctors felt pressured to act before there was reasonable diagnostic certainty. Guidelines regarding this "four-hour rule" have been relaxed, but we still have no idea whether any such rule is helpful.

The second example of an unproven systems intervention coming into question is the use of "door-to-balloon time" as an incentivized quality marker. From the late 1990s to the very early 2000s, observational studies showed that when patients come to the emergency room with a heart attack, time matters. The specific time that mattered was the time from when the patient walked into the ER to the time when the blocked artery

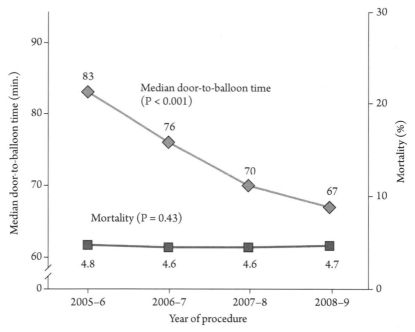

5.1 Declining door-to-balloon times without associated declines in mortality.
Source: Menees DS, Peterson ED, Wang Y, et al., Door-to-balloon time and mortality among patients undergoing primary PCI. N Engl J Med. 2013;369:901–909. Copyright © 2013, Massachusetts Medical Society. Used with permission from the Massachusetts Medical Society.

was opened by a balloon deployed by an interventional cardiologist. We call this time "reperfusion time." Opening arteries in a timely fashion makes perfect sense, and it is associated with better outcomes. There is, however, an important difference between saying that patients who undergo timely reperfusion do well and saying we ought to create a national campaign to improve reperfusion times. By 2006, however, we were well into the latter—a massive initiative to bring the slowest hospitals up to grade.

In 2013 a study was published that raised doubts about our efforts. The study found that between 2005 and 2009, door-to-balloon times were reduced across the nation; the number of patients waiting longer than 90 minutes decreased from 40.3 percent to 16.9 percent. Unfortunately, mortality was completely unchanged over this time period. Figure 5.1 displays in a striking way the decline in door-to-balloon time graphed against the unchanging mortality. Our tremendous and costly efforts improved door-to-balloon time but did not yield improvements in survival.

· Why was the intervention to reduce door-to-balloon time ineffective? There are several possible, but only speculative, explanations. The first is that we were wrong all along that door-to-balloon time matters. Maybe a shorter door-to-balloon time is unimportant in and of itself but is a marker of better hospitals that do everything better. This is akin to noting that lawyers who wear Armani suits win more court cases. An intervention to clothe more lawyers in Armani would be unlikely to improve the performance of the better-suited attorneys. Another explanation is that door-to-balloon time is not all that matters. Logically, you would think the time from symptom onset (which happens at home) to balloon is what matters and that (emergency room) door-to-balloon is just one part of this. By this logic, we are not targeting the right metric. We need people to respond faster to their symptoms, 911 systems to run more efficiently, and ambulances to move faster. Lastly, decreasing door-to-balloon time might be an example of diminishing returns. Going from 180 minutes to 120 minutes provides a large benefit, 120 to 100 may also make a difference, but going from 99 to 90 minutes does not matter all that much. A final possibility—one that proponents of the intervention favor—is that door-to-balloon time reductions did help, but, over time, sicker people underwent the procedure. While it looks like no net improvement, the reality is that everyone is improving, and people are benefiting who previously did not even receive the procedure. The truth is that we do not know which explanation is right. Only a randomized trial can tell us whether or not asking hospitals to reduce their door-to-balloon time saves lives. Instead, door-to-balloon-time efforts were widely implemented and remain untested. Of course, it must be acknowledged that the study we describe is not the final word on the subject, but it does highlight a not-uncommon outcome of systems interventions—whether proved or disproved, they cost society billions of dollars.

THE SCIENCE OF SYSTEMS

We end with a major and conclusive reversal of a systems intervention. In 2001 a randomized controlled trial found that using insulin to lower patients' blood-sugar levels to normal levels could improve survival in a surgical intensive care unit. This intervention was more novel than it might seem, because one of the body's responses to critical illness is actually to raise blood-sugar levels. This trial was not of the highest level. It was a single-center study and was unblinded (more about that in chapter 9). In 2006 the same center reproduced the results in patients in the medical intensive care units. Professional societies embraced the strict blood-sugar targets, and entire hospitals instituted quality interventions aimed at meeting and enforcing the strict standard.

Fortunately, this systems intervention was ultimately rigorously tested. In 2009 a multicenter (42-hospital) randomized trial of more than 6,000 patients tested the intensive blood-sugar-control strategy against a more permissive one. This study found that strict blood-sugar reduction actually increased deaths by 2.6 percentage points at 90 days. This dramatic result meant that for every 40 patients treated with the intensive strategy, a patient died.

The story of blood-sugar control in the ICU is a classic in the medical-reversal genre. It is a story of poorly designed studies, single-center trials, and surrogate end points. We include it here, in our discussion of systems interventions, because as clinicians who worked in hospitals during the years the intervention was embraced, we remember the efforts hospitals made to ensure the strict target was met. Nurses received special training, pharmacies were ready to keep insulin running, and it was on the daily checklist of ICU rounds. In the end, all this effort helped no one and hurt a few.

These days we hear statements like: "The 20th century was about the science of medicine; the 21st will be about the science of systems" and "The major problem in medicine is to take what we know and ensure it gets done right." These catchy phrases might be true, but so far it seems that when it comes to systems interventions, we have failed to learn the lessons of reversals taught by medical and surgical interventions gone awry. Systems interventions are often adopted based on scant evidence, and when this happens, they are probably just as likely to be overturned as any other medical treatment—no matter how much sense they seem to make. Being on the losing end of a systems intervention is just as bad as being treated with a medication that is later shown to be ineffective or harmful.

6
FINDING FLAWED THERAPIES ON OUR OWN

THE PRECEDING CHAPTERS have been pretty hard on doctors. The one thing every practice we discussed had in common is that they were recommended by physicians or performed under their guidance. These examples show that, despite years of training and the best intentions, doctors often recommend treatments that do not work. We like to think of this review less as an opportunity to scold our profession and more as a reminder to be humble. Before we move on from our long list of reversals, let us leave doctors' offices and hospitals and go into our homes. As it turns out, we do not need doctors to suggest flawed therapies; we do quite well finding them all by ourselves.

William Osler, easily the most quoted physician of the 20th century, wrote, "The desire to take medicine is perhaps the greatest feature which distinguishes man from animals." By this measure, we are becoming progressively more human. Americans use more self-prescribed treatments every year. These treatments come in many forms. There are vitamins and minerals, dietary supplements, and procedures of all kinds—acupuncture, chiropractic manipulation, and intravenous vitamin therapy, to name just a few. Many of these interventions either have no evidence supporting their

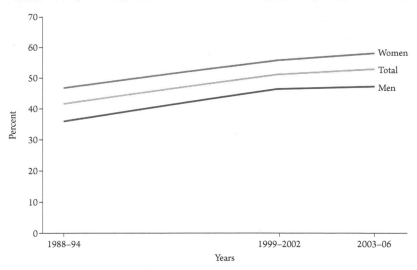

6.1 Percentage of adults using dietary supplements. *Source:* Centers for Disease Control and Prevention, www.cdc.gov/nchs/data/databriefs/db61.htm.

benefit (and are thus potentially open to reversal) or have already been shown to be ineffective. For clarity, throughout this chapter we will refer to these self-prescribed remedies as complementary and refer to those directly sanctioned and prescribed by doctors as traditional.

We are all particularly susceptible to these sorts of complementary treatments. A recent survey by the Centers for Disease Control and Prevention revealed that more than half of all Americans use some sort of dietary supplement. The survey results are displayed graphically in figure 6.1. We admit that a search through our own medicine cabinets revealed two or three of these products (or at least did before we researched this chapter). What is so important about the reversals that involve complementary treatments is that they potentially affect a huge number of people. To be affected by the reversals that we dwelled on in the past few chapters, you had to have a disease and then see a doctor who chose to prescribe an unsubstantiated treatment. Even the screening tests we discussed only affect people for whom the test is recommended, and then only if they seek it out. By definition, the complementary therapies we discuss below are available to anyone and everyone.

To reflect the ubiquity of these treatments, instead of using one of our patients as an example, we will use a friend. Joanne happily volunteered the details of her case, though she did ask us to change her name.

Joanne knows that some of what she does probably does not make much of a difference. She eats low-fat cottage cheese and yogurt even though she has heard that reduced-fat dairy products may be no better for you than the luxurious full-fat versions. She uses low-fat salad dressing and almond milk. At this point she cannot even remember why, but she figures they help keep her weight down. She makes sure to have a glass of red wine and a small square of dark chocolate each night—she says these are good for her heart, but she also smiles when she says this. She eats only brown rice. She briefly followed a low-carb and then a gluten-free diet, but those interventions were too painful to last long. She is pretty sure that she has heard about data, at one time or another, supporting all these dietary quirks, but she is also pretty sure that she has heard data suggesting the opposite.

Joanne is more confident about some of her other health habits. She takes a multivitamin, specially balanced for women, every day. She also takes calcium and vitamin D, daily. She is 57, after all, and although she has no reason to think she has osteoporosis, a little extra boost for her bones cannot hurt. She also takes glucosamine because her knees feel a bit creaky these days and (with prompting) admits to having once visited an acupuncture practitioner for the same pain. When she is sick, she uses echinacea to speed her recovery.

Like most Americans, Joanne has chosen a range of practices in pursuit of health. Like many of us, she admits to being a little confused. She has heard various practices supported at one time or by one news source while the same practice is dismissed as ineffective, or even harmful, at another time or by another source. One day fat is the enemy, the next it is sugar. In January you are supposed to do aerobic exercise; in February weight-training is in vogue. Studies extol the virtues of blackberries one week and peaches the next.

The story of how products and procedures become popular complementary health practices is interesting and a nice prelude to future chapters in which we delve into the causes of reversals in medicine. But before we get into that story, let us specifically consider some of Joanne's chosen interventions and why they should be considered reversals.

To begin, we will limit the discussion to the "interventions" Joanne has chosen and steer away from her diet. Joanne says that these interventions are the things in which she is most confident. She began using a multivitamin after learning that the body needs a small quantity of a wide range of vitamins and minerals to thrive. She believes these are important because she thinks she does not "eat right." She began the calcium and vitamin D after menopause to improve the strength of her bones. Her mother had a knee replacement, so the glucosamine seemed like a no-brainer as a preventive therapy. She tried acupuncture in an effort to stay away from pharmaceutical painkillers. The echinacea just works for colds. Period.

REVERSALS

Let's start with the clear reversals. Glucosamine and chondroitin are a part of normal, healthy cartilage and are marketed to promote healthy joints. In using one of these, Joanne is in good company. As of 2004, more than $700 million was spent on glucosamine, chondroitin sulfate, or combination pills. In 2006 a trial randomized more than 1,500 people to one of five treatments. The treatments were glucosamine, chondroitin, a combination of the glucosamine and chondroitin, an anti-inflammatory drug, and a placebo. At the end of the study, there was no difference in improvement in pain among the people who took glucosamine, chondroitin, the combination, or the placebo. In 2010, researchers looking at data from 10 different trials concluded that neither glucosamine, chondroitin, nor their combination improve joint pain.

How about echinacea? When it comes to treating the common cold, there are no proven therapies. This reality is the foundation for many dubious claims. Nearly 20 percent of Americans report having used echinacea in the past 30 days. Like Joanne, many use the medication to reduce the duration of cold symptoms. In 2005 researchers randomly assigned volunteers to echinacea or placebo and then exposed them to the cold virus. (We assume the volunteers were well compensated.) They found that echinacea did not reduce the duration of symptoms among patients who contracted a cold. These results were later supported by an analysis of seven randomized trials, only one of which found that echinacea reduced the duration of cold symptoms when compared to a placebo. (In the same analysis, the authors examined 12 studies that looked at using echinacea to prevent colds; none of these studies showed an effect.)

Acupuncture dates back more than 3,000 years. It is a popular treatment for pain and has been advocated for ailments as diverse as Bell's palsy and nicotine addiction. Recently, acupuncture has been studied relentlessly. These studies have included some beautifully designed trials in which acupuncture was compared to sham acupuncture (either using toothpicks, instead of real needles, or retracting acupuncture needles). A recent, and impressive, effort to bring together all this research analyzed any review of the acupuncture literature that was published between 2000 and 2009. The authors searched for reviews indexed in databases of the Western, Chinese, and Korean scientific literature. In the end, the authors concluded that there is "little truly convincing evidence that acupuncture is effective in reducing pain." They also enumerated a few examples of acupuncture causing real harm.

Because of the ubiquity of multivitamin use, no topic is more controversial than this one. The reasons people take vitamins are varied. Like Joanne, they may take them because they feel their diet is inadequate, or they may hope the supplement will decrease their chances of having heart disease or cancer, or improve their longevity. In 2009 an observational study of postmenopausal women was done. This trial studied 161,808 women, who were enrolled in observational or randomized trials. Over 40 percent of these women had chosen to take multivitamins. The use of multivitamins was not associated with declines in cancer, heart disease, stroke, or mortality. However, this was an observational study, which, as we have seen, can mislead us (see chapter 10 for more on observational studies). In this case, however, randomized trials confirm the lack of benefit. In 2013, the latest and most extensive review of the randomized trials that have studied multivitamin use found no clear benefit on overall survival, heart disease, or cancer. The *Annals of Internal Medicine*, the journal that published this study, published an article in the same issue entitled, "Enough Is Enough: Stop Wasting Money on Vitamin and Mineral Supplements."

Finally, we come to calcium and vitamin D, which Joanne takes to strengthen her bones. If multivitamins are the most controversial, calcium supplementation is probably the most confusing. Our bones are made of calcium, and vitamin D helps our body absorb calcium. In youth, adequate calcium intake is crucial as we build our skeletons. As adults, many people do not achieve the recommended intake of calcium and vitamin D—1,000 mg. of calcium and 600 international units of vitamin D daily, the equivalent of about 4 servings of dairy products. For years, the common practice among American women (a practice endorsed by countless physicians and several professional groups) was to supplement inadequate dietary intake. If you only have two servings of dairy, take a calcium and vitamin D tablet to make up the deficit. This recommendation made sense for a couple of reasons. Unlike most vitamins, if you do not consume enough calcium, doctors cannot easily detect a deficit with a blood test. Your body works hard to maintain a normal calcium level—if calcium intake is low, your blood calcium level is maintained at the expense of your bones. Also, fracture among elderly women is often a devastating injury; why not do something to try to prevent it?

Unfortunately, supplementing calcium and vitamin D seems to not help. Similar to the stories above, recent analyses of randomized trials find that calcium and vitamin D supplementation does not reduce the risk of fractures among healthy women. For this reason, the U.S. Preventive Services Task Force (USPSTF) now recommends against the supplements.*

For years we have known that calcium and vitamin D supplementation has an important adverse effect: an increase in kidney stones. In 2010 a group of researchers identified another potential side effect: heart attacks. Initially, they found that calcium supplementation (without vitamin D) actually increased a woman's chance of having a heart attack. At that time, many argued that the increased risk was seen because calcium was being given without vitamin D. In 2011 the same group examined studies of vitamin D plus calcium, and again they found the risk of heart attack was elevated in women who took the supplements. In short, all the recent evidence argues that calcium and vitamin D supplementation probably does not improve the outcome for which it is intended but probably does increase the risk of an even more serious health outcome. Healthy women should not take this supplement.

Before we attempt to explain why we seem to be so attracted to complementary therapies, it is worth clarifying our use of the word *reversal*. By now, you see that not all reversals are created equal. The common thread among all medical reversals is that a large, well-done study—typically a randomized controlled trial—finds no benefit (or finds that harms outweigh any benefits that do exist) for a common practice. The reason a practice was adopted in the first place varies widely. For some practices, we had laboratory experiments, observational trials, or surrogate end points

---

* Currently, the USPSTF also says there is insufficient evidence to argue for, or against, higher doses. Calcium and vitamin D probably do help older women living in nursing homes and those who already have osteoporosis.

that supported their use. In this chapter, we have discussed therapies that gained traction based on little more than anecdotal testimonies. It is tempting to conclude that some reversals are worse than others, and that the missteps doctors make are somehow more understandable because they are based on science, albeit flawed science. By the end of this book, we believe that, like us, you will reject this conclusion. Having studied hundreds of reversals, we do not think that, on average, doctors have higher standards than other people. Many medical practices are adopted based on studies as flawed as those for herbal supplements. Ultimately, it really does not matter how many pieces of evidence support a practice—all that matters is the quality of the evidence. With that clarification, let's turn to our psychology.

WHY WE TAKE WHAT WE TAKE

So if that is the evidence, why do Joanne and so many of us use these complementary treatments? The adoption of these therapies seems to follow a well-worn route, one that is not dissimilar to that taken by more traditional medical therapies. Most therapies begin with an engaging story or history. Complementary therapies satisfy some need that traditional medical therapies do not. These therapies do not rise to prominence unassisted. There are usually influential supporters and people positioned to profit from their adoption helping them along. In the United States, complementary treatments get a passive assist from the federal government in that, unlike the highly regulated traditional therapies, there is no requirement of proof that they are effective. Lastly, and in this way they are not dissimilar from traditional therapies, when the effectiveness of these complementary treatments is rigorously tested and they are proven ineffective, these treatments are not readily abandoned.

So let us follow the twists and turns along the road to acceptance for a few common complementary therapies. The road begins with a story that makes the treatment appealing. The story usually involves a long history of use, some "natural origin," and a reason that the treatment should work. Glucosamine is a natural component of cartilage, so its ingestion should certainly benefit our joints, whose function is so dependent on cartilage. Vitamins and minerals are, by definition, substances that our body can neither synthesize nor live without. In addition, there are frightening medical syndromes caused by their absence. The fact that in today's industrialized world we never see rickets, scurvy, pellagra, or other vitamin-deficiency syndromes in healthy people with anything remotely resembling a reasonable diet does not dissuade people from assuming the necessity of supplements. If you want a sense of how rare these syndromes are now, ask your doctor to describe the symptoms of pellagra or beriberi—and prepare for an uncomfortable silence.

Some accepted alternative therapies lack modern physiological explanations of their utility and rely on historical precedent. Few accept the explanation that acupuncture corrects imbalances in the flow of qi through our meridians. Instead, its history of use over thousands of years is convincing. Echinacea's use for diverse medicinal purposes by Plains Indians accounts for some of the faith in its power over the common cold.

Every complementary therapy makes up for some shortcoming created by the culture and practice of 21st-century medicine. The great successes of modern medicine and public health have been to control the diseases that suddenly and tragically strike down people in their youth. Infant mortality has seen unimaginable declines, and few of us spend time worrying about dying of polio, tuberculosis, or influenza, let alone appendicitis or gallstones. These successes leave us to worry about the diseases of aging—those diseases that set in motion the unavoidable and inexorable decline to death. Since the best medicine can do is "decrease your risk" or perhaps "delay" the development of cancers and heart disease, we are left to fend for ourselves with alternative therapies. Add to this the progressively depersonalized nature of medicine. When a visit to your doctor means spending 15 minutes with an overworked physician, one who tries to keep to an impossibly busy schedule by documenting your visit in her computer while you talk, it is not surprising that people look to an acupuncture provider who might spend an hour talking to you while actually touching your body.

Complementary therapies do not reach the shelves of GNC by a magical, organic process. Some of these therapies are backed by famous thinkers. Vitamins famously got their boost from Linus Pauling, a brilliant scientist and winner of two Nobel prizes, who spent his later years promoting megadoses of vitamins, based on theory alone. If other therapies are not backed by a prize-winning scientist, there are celebrities, celebrity doctors, and companies anxious to be a part of this $27 billion industry. Every day you can turn on the television or radio and find a celebrity physician or a guest on a talk show discussing a new complementary remedy. Dr. Mehmet Oz was called before Congress to explain his exuberant endorsement of unproven supplements. Many magazines fill their pages with "healthful tips" to keep you feeling or looking healthier or younger. These are the complementary therapies we are discussing. These topics draw viewers and help television and radio shows, magazines, and websites sell advertising.

An interesting fact about vitamins and supplements in the United States is that they can be marketed without any of the rigorous testing that is necessary for prescription and over-the-counter drugs.* While makers of traditional medications and devices must demonstrate their products' safety and efficacy to the FDA before they go on the market, supplements, defined as substances intended to provide nutrients that might otherwise not be consumed in sufficient quantities, need only to be safe. This difference makes supplements, when they are used to treat or prevent disease, terrifically prone to reversal—there is usually little or no evidence that they work. One of the few places to find information about the effectiveness of supplements is the National Institutes of Health's National Center for Complementary and Alternative Medicine (NCCAM). NCCAM's website is one of our favorite places to while away a few hours. Because the federal government does not regulate supplements, the frequently negative findings described on this site are only informational and do not affect labeling or marketing of these products.

We are at the final stop on the road toward acceptance for complementary therapies. This is where these therapies, as sometimes happens, are reversed. In general, as we will learn in chapter 8, medicine is slow to abandon therapies that are proved ineffective. Available evidence suggests that the lay population is even slower to abandon ineffective therapies than the medical field—in fact, we seem to be totally unaffected by negative data. We have already seen that vitamin use has increased recently, this in the setting of mounting evidence that it has no beneficial effect. As for acupuncture, in 1997 there were 27 visits to an acupuncturist for every 1,000 adults in the United States; in 2007 the number was 79. Why is this the case? Part of the increase may be explained by cognitive dissonance.

Cognitive dissonance is the psychological theory that proposes that we have difficulty making sense of information that contradicts our

* For a terrific recent discussion of the regulation of "conventional" and "alternative" therapies, we point you to Paul Offit's book *Do You Believe in Magic?* (HarperCollins, 2013).

worldview. Imagine a person who understands that a treatment—a vitamin, say, or a procedure that he chooses and pays for—has risks and benefits. He decides to give it a try and begins to feel better, or at least not worse. He tends to believe that this treatment, in which he has invested money and time, is beneficial. Later, if he is told that the procedure never worked, this creates dissonance. People often respond to such dissonance by more fervently believing that the treatment does work, and that the critics of it are wrong. If you buy a car that you love and the axle breaks after two weeks, you are more likely to blame those darn potholes than the lemon you bought.

WHAT TO EAT

Let's get back to Joanne, whom we have probably picked on enough. Joanne was actually pretty comfortable with her choices of vitamins and supplements, but she felt hopelessly confused about her attempts to eat a healthful diet. We think she is right to feel confused. Each week we read stories about the healthfulness of the food we eat that are hard to believe, or we hear stories that explicitly contradict stories we heard last week. Where can we find some certainty about dietary recommendations?

The PREDIMED trial (Prevención con Dieta Mediterránea) was a study published in the *New England Journal of Medicine* in 2013. A multicenter trial conducted in Spain, PREDIMED randomly assigned more than 7,000 patients at high risk for a cardiovascular event to either a Mediterranean diet supplemented with extra virgin olive oil or nuts, or a control diet.* The Mediterranean diet even sounded palatable: 4 tablespoons of extra virgin olive oil a day, at least seven glasses of wine each week for those so inclined, and no calorie counting. The diet did discourage soft drinks, commercial bakery goods, sweets, pastries, spreadable fats, and red or processed meats. After about five years the trial was stopped, because there were fewer strokes in the Mediterranean diet groups. This is one of the few times a randomized trial of a dietary intervention showed a benefit for this kind of end point. Most diets are never tested in a randomized trial, and when they are, the main outcome of the study is usually short-term weight loss. Still, in PREDIMED, if you looked at mortality, there was no difference between

---

* The trial enrolled men between 55 and 80 and women between 60 and 80, who had either diabetes or three cardiac risk factors.

the diets. Even the reduction in strokes was small. You had to treat about 90 people with the diet for five years to prevent one stroke.

Given the flow of this book, you probably think that we are telling you about PREDIMED because it was later contradicted. It was not. We are writing about it because it shows just how difficult it is to do a study of a diet that proves anything. Even when you take thousands of people— people who, because of their age and medical conditions are at risk for bad outcomes—and randomize them to a diet, and get them to stick with it, and follow them for years, and find a statistically significant difference, the end result is still very, very small. And even if you think this one dietary intervention is worth it, what about adding sushi to your diet, just one meal a week? What about cooking Indian lentils and rice? How about eating a little kimchi?

When you start to think about the breadth of dietary options—even just diets typically associated with healthy living—homemade Italian or Indian or Greek or Japanese or Chinese food—you start to realize that there will never be enough trials to answer all the questions. Furthermore, when you think about how to test diets for people in their thirties and forties, you realize you would have to follow even greater numbers of people for even longer periods of time to see if any diet has a survival benefit. We would need such large studies, of so many combinations, over so many years, that we would run out of people to randomize. For this reason, it is unlikely we will ever have the set of randomized trials we need to guide the dietary choices of those who are well.

So how about observational studies? Diet may be one place where all we have to go on are observational trials. As Joanne noted at the beginning of the chapter, however, observational studies often contradict other observational trials. Plus, as we will see in chapter 9, researchers can conduct so many analyses in an observational study that, when it comes to dietary habits, studies are less like science and more like an opinion poll. To illustrate the absurdity of observational research on nutrition, two researchers randomly selected 50 ingredients from a cookbook. They found articles reporting cancer risk associated with 40 of the ingredients. Their conclusion was well stated in the study's title, "Is Everything We Eat Associated with Cancer?" The message is clear—when it comes to nutrition, you can get observational studies to say anything.

Given these sobering facts, what is a healthy diet? And how should you eat? Both of us are partial to arguments made and defended at length elsewhere. For instance, Michael Pollan has provided a reasonable framework and set of rules to guide healthy eating in his books *In Defense of Food* and *The Omnivore's Dilemma*. He agrees that women like Joanne are right to feel frustrated. His statements like, "Eat food, mostly plants, and not too much" and "Don't eat anything your great-grandmother wouldn't recognize as food," seem like good advice. Of course, we would add: be skeptical of any nutritional claims; they are unlikely to be from randomized trials and may soon be proved wrong.

CONCLUSION

So what have we learned? Laypeople, just like doctors, are prone to adopt therapies that are not well founded. Unfortunately, many of the therapies do not actually help us—and some may even do harm. Not long after you read this page, you will be presented a new complementary remedy. The treatment will be backed by a good story and maybe even a physiological explanation of how and why it will help. It will be supported by someone who has a stake in it—someone who needs to sell advertising on a show or in a magazine or someone who needs to keep the product moving from health-food store shelves. Some of these treatments might even make us feel better—though only for a short time and only because we hoped and expected that they would.

Our goal for the future of complementary health care is reasonable, although it might also be grand. We hope that people will hold the treatments they choose for themselves to the same standard to which doctors *should* hold the treatments they prescribe for their patients. If we ever reach this point, we will not have to decide between traditional and complementary therapies; we will just choose therapies that we know work.

7

THE FREQUENCY OF MEDICAL REVERSAL

WE HAVE SEEN THAT REVERSAL OCCURS in all aspects of medicine. Whether the medical intervention is a pill, a procedure, a surgery, a diagnostic test, a screening campaign, or even a checklist that doctors or nurses follow, all sorts of medical practices have been found not to work. When the two of us first began thinking and writing about reversal, peer reviewers at medical journals were surprised by our argument. Sure, they conceded, occasionally a medical practice fails, and when that happens it is certainly memorable. But, they added, those are exceptional cases; most of what doctors do is sound. And so a question was born. How often does medical reversal happen? Is it rare but memorable—like an earthquake in California? Or is it ubiquitous—like snowstorms during a Chicago winter? We were fascinated by the question and intrigued by how best to answer it.

In an ideal world, the way to measure reversal would be to make a list of all existing standards of care. (This would be a very long list. It would include everything that doctors do.) Every practice that was based on strong evidence, that had bettered a lesser therapy in a well-done randomized controlled trial (or more than one), would get a pass. Everything that remained would be tested in rigorous trials to see if it worked. Practices that came out ahead in those trials would also get a pass; those that didn't would be identified as a case of medical reversal (and, more importantly, would no longer be offered to patients).

Of course, we do not live in an ideal world. Quantifying everything that would need to be tested would, in itself, be a career's work. The cost of trials to test every unproven therapy would probably consume the entirety of the global research budget. So we tried to devise another way to measure it. One thought was to examine the treatments that were developed during a specific time interval, say 1995 to 2000, and ask what percentage was shown not to work by 2010. A nice idea, but also flawed, since most medical practices were not reexamined between 2000 and 2010. Because only a small fraction of the standards of care would be tested, we would underestimate the frequency of medical reversal.

Another way to answer the question would be to look at all clinical trials published during some time interval that tested standards of care and ask how many contradict those standards. Unfortunately, despite the growing databases of clinical trials, there is no easy way to get a list of such studies and their results. Besides, most trials that test a standard of care test trivial comparisons: is it better to give steroid injections for osteoarthritis of the knee every three months or every six months; do antacid medicines work better when taken once a day in double dose or twice a day in single dose? Instead, we were interested in trials that test fundamental questions: do steroid injections or antacids work at all? Is an established medical practice better than an older, proven one? Is it better than no treatment at all?

Finally, we devised a way to estimate reversal. Like the others, it had its flaws but it was practical and would give us some interesting data. We would review every article in the most prestigious and highest-impact medical journal, the *New England Journal of Medicine (NEJM)*, in a single year. NEJM papers typically ask important questions. We would analyze any study that tested a current standard of care. Because hundreds of articles are published annually in NEJM, we picked 2009, the last complete year at the time of our investigation, in order to make the task manageable. As we worked on our project, we surveyed the literature to see if others had tried to estimate the incidence of medical reversal in the medical literature. Of the millions of papers published in medical journals, only one came close to what we envisioned.

In 2005 John Ioannidis, a physician-researcher and a truly innovative thinker, wanted to measure what proportion of important findings in med-icine were later contradicted. His strategy was to start with highly cited works. These were studies that were referenced more than 1,000 times by other publications. These are the papers that really influence the practice of medicine. (It is the goal of pretty much every medical researcher to pen such an influential paper.) Ioannidis considered all the highly cited papers published in key medical journals during the years 1990 to 2003. Of those, 45 found that a medical intervention was effective. He then tracked all reports of these interventions' efficacy over the years to come. He found that seven (16 percent) were later found to be ineffective, another seven (16 percent) were found less effective than initially believed, 20 (44 per-cent) were supported in future studies, and 11 (24 percent) were never tested again. The practices that were later found to be ineffective included the use of vitamins to prevent cancer and heart disease, treatment of over-whelming infections, and the use of nitric oxide in critically ill patients.

The study suggested that 16 percent of the most widely cited medical lit-erature is later contradicted. Although an interesting and beautifully done study, it did not answer our particular question. We wanted to know what percentage of what doctors actually do is wrong. Not just the topics that get a lot of buzz (and citations), like cancer prevention and heart disease, but even the unsung heroes in medicine—treating back pain, rashes, or Bell's palsy.

In 2011, with the help of Victor Gall, who at the time was a bright medi-cal student at Northwestern University, we published our results in a paper entitled "The Frequency of Medical Reversal." Not surprisingly, we found that most research in the NEJM, 77 percent in fact, concerned new medical practices and not standards of care. Of the 35 studies that did examine the current standards of care, 16 (46 percent) showed that the standard of care was ineffective. These were medical reversals. Standard therapy was no bet-ter than either the previous standard or no treatment at all.

Like good researchers (and ones always looking for another entry on the curriculum vitae) we set out to extend our findings. Our next project was to increase the time span that we studied from 1 year to 10. With the help of 10 colleagues—it was a pretty big job—we reviewed 2,044 origi-nal articles published in the NEJM between 2001 and 2010. Of these, 363 articles reported the results of studies that tested the efficacy of an estab-lished practice. Reversals were found in 146 (40 percent) of these studies,

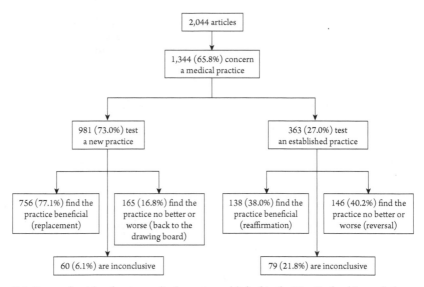

7.1 Types of articles about a medical practice published in the *New England Journal of Medicine* between 2001 and 2010.

138 (38 percent) of the studies reaffirmed the benefit of the new practice, and 79 (22 percent) were inconclusive. The breakdown of these results is shown graphically in figure 7.1.

Forty percent is a lot. Nearly half of what doctors do. If that much of medical practice is ineffective, it is pretty scary. The number did fit with how we felt about the medicine we see practiced every day and the medical literature we have followed during our careers. But the number really does not tell the whole story. First, for some fields of medicine, those for which the evidence base is weak, an estimate that 40 percent of standard therapy is ineffective is probably about right (or maybe even low). For other fields, those in which new therapies tend to be rigorously tested, the proportion that is ineffective is probably smaller. Second, the proportion of practice that is suspect depends on how a doctor practices. We know doctors, in every field, who do everything that is reasonable and evidence-based and no more. We also know doctors who test the limits of reason daily. So the average may not apply to your doctor (or any one doctor).

Of course, not everyone was happy with our findings, and some quibbled with the exact number. We agreed with some of the criticism. We may have overestimated the prevalence of reversal, because the NEJM likes to publish controversial papers and may therefore gravitate to papers that report the overturning of a standard. Then again, testing the standard of care is provocative because it happens so rarely. The NEJM publishes plenty of papers that validate what doctors do. In our analysis, they published about the same number of studies that validated current practice as they did studies that overturned it.

We may also have underestimated the frequency of reversal. By and large, doctors do not test their own standard of care. Doctors are doing what they believe is best for their patients. It takes an innovative and brave researcher (and a bit of a contrarian) to test a practice to which most of her colleagues are committed. There is also the issue of money. There is little incentive to attempt to overturn a practice from which you are profiting. Not many orthopedists would be willing to investigate whether joint replacement is better than a sham procedure. They believe in the procedure and are making a handsome profit from it. The manufacturers of the prosthetic hip are even less likely to fund such a study. Thus, countless trials are not done.

But in an important way, the number does not even matter. Earthquakes are rare in California, for sure, but we still build office towers and houses strong enough to withstand them. As long as reversal is not rare (and our data argue very strongly that it is not) and affects human health, we should address it. Doctors understand that what they do is beneficial for patients on average but not necessarily for the individual patient. (We discuss this further in chapter 9.) The data on medical reversal, however, suggest that much of what we believe helps a subset of a population may actually help no one.

Whether the actual number is a little higher or a little lower, it does fit nicely with the old adage "Half of what you are taught in medical school is wrong. The trouble is, we do not know which half."

So although our results are limited, coming from a small slice of published literature, which itself is a small slice of what researchers think are plausible questions to ask and test, they do tell us that medical reversal is not rare. Many of the reversals we discovered have been outlined in the previous chapters. Reversals included medical therapies (prednisone use among preschool-aged children with viral wheezing and cholesterol-lowering drugs for patients on dialysis), a checklist (to assure tight glycemic control in intensive-care-unit patients), invasive procedures (percutaneous intervention for atherosclerotic renal artery disease), and screening tests (prostate cancer screening). In a review of research from a single journal, there was an example of medical reversal from virtually every corner of modern medicine. In the appendix, we give a short summary of every article that we interpreted as a reversal in this study. Experts may not agree with every one of our conclusions—sometimes arguing that the overturned therapy was not really an accepted standard or that the reversal was not complete. We ourselves had some heated discussions about what should and should not make the list. The important thing about the list is that even if you might quibble with an inclusion (or exclusion) or two, the weight of the overall number is great.

As is often the case when a topic is important, many researchers get interested in it at the same time and examine it in their own way. While we were completing our work, we began to see a lot of similar findings appearing in the literature. A project of the *British Medical Journal Clinical Evidence* completed a review of 3,000 medical practices. Those researchers found that 35 percent of medical practices are effective (or likely to be effective); 15 percent are harmful, unlikely to be beneficial, or a tradeoff between benefits and harms; and 50 percent are of unknown effectiveness.

How do these findings square with our results? Quite nicely, it turns out. The *Clinical Evidence* project maps the landscape of all medical practices. Some work, some do not (these are reversals still stuck in a lag time before doctors abandon them), and for some we simply do not have enough information. Our results apply to this last group; the 50 percent of practices about which we do not have adequate information. Our research suggests that, if you subjected the untested 50 percent to real scrutiny, 40 percent of these would be found to be, at best, ineffective. Our work shrinks the gray zone (actually the hatched area) of figure 7.2.

In a similar vein, a team in Australia screened 5,209 articles in an effort to find medical practices that were unlikely to be of any benefit to patients. The results, published in 2012, listed 156 potentially ineffective or unsafe practices. There was some overlap with practices that we identified in our work. The Australian group cited eight practices that we included in our catalog of reversals. Among these were the use of arthroscopic surgery for knee osteoarthritis, endovascular repair of some abdominal aortic aneurysms, and amnioinfusion for high-risk pregnant women. While it is a bit surprising that there was not more overlap with our work, the Australians

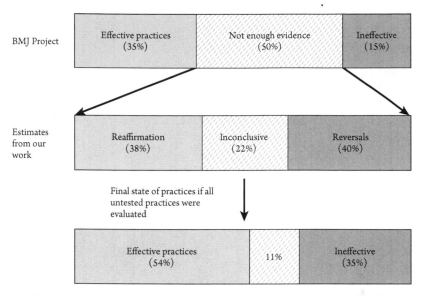

7.2 Combining the BMJ *Clinical Evidence* project with our work on the frequency of medical reversal.

looked at the entire body of medical practice, while we looked at 10 years of trials in one journal. In the end, our study added well over 100 practices to the Australians' already impressive list.

During the past few years, researchers have produced multiple pieces of evidence supporting the idea that there is much that doctors do that is, at least, unproved. When these practices are examined, a sizable subset is found to be ineffective, when compared to previous practices. Some of the practices are actually found to be harmful. The obvious questions that need to be answered are, Why is reversal so common? and, What can be done to make it less so?

8

THE HARMS OF MEDICAL REVERSAL

:: TODAY'S PATIENTS, TOMORROW'S PATIENTS,
AND THE HEALTH-CARE FIELD

WHEN ANITA KRAMER WOKE UP, she could not move her left arm. She tried to speak, but her words were garbled. She panicked and thought, "This can't be happening." She somehow managed to call 911. The emergency dispatcher initially had trouble understanding her but eventually recognized the symptoms. He told her to take an aspirin and sent an ambulance. Anita had just had a stroke.

By now, most of us recognize the basic signs of stroke. Nationwide campaigns have increased the awareness of the common symptoms with the hope that people will receive treatment as quickly as possible. Strokes occur when the brain is deprived of oxygenated blood. Sometimes a stroke is caused by a narrowed artery impairing blood flow to the area of the brain beyond the obstruction. More often, a cholesterol plaque or blood clot breaks off from the wall of an artery and clogs a more distant vessel.

Because Anita woke up with symptoms, her doctors in the emergency room are in a jam. They do not know if the stroke occurred 30 minutes before, when she woke up, or at midnight the night before. This would not be important were it not that our most effective treatment for strokes, tissue plasminogen activator, or TPA, only works when given within about four and half hours of the onset of symptoms. TPA works by breaking up clots. The drug is such a powerful blood thinner that its risks (including lethal hemorrhage) aren't trivial. After four and half hours, the risks of the drug begin to outweigh its benefit.

With TPA off the table, there are really no options to treat the stroke. Fortunately, with time and physical therapy, many patients will recover at least some of their lost abilities. All of the evaluation and treatment that Anita will receive in the hospital will be intended to decrease her risk of having another stroke. She receives atorvastatin to lower her cholesterol and a combination of aspirin and dipyridamole to thin her blood. Her doctors monitor her heart rhythm, looking for atrial fibrillation, a common cardiac arrhythmia that increases the risk for stroke. They also look at her heart for the presence of blood clots. If either of these is detected, she will need to be on another class of blood thinners. (We used to look for a defect between two chambers of the heart, which could allow blood clots from the legs to travel to the brain. We do not [or should not] do this anymore, because a major trial showed that closing this hole was not beneficial— another example of medical reversal, which we will leave for another day.) The doctors look at the carotid arteries, usually with ultrasound. A buildup of cholesterol plaque in these large vessels in the neck can be surgically repaired, markedly decreasing the risk of future stroke. And, for the past decade, many physicians have looked for narrowing of the smaller vessels in the brain. If one of these was narrowed, we could reopen it with a stent (just as we do for arteries in the heart). The idea was that this procedure could decrease the risk of future strokes.

During Anita's evaluation, her doctors discovered that she had a 70 percent stenosis (narrowing) in the middle cerebral artery, a major blood vessel of the brain. Her neurologist recommended a stent. Anita got the stent. Six days later, she had another stroke that left her more disabled than the first.

In 2011, 10 years after this practice began and 6 years after the stent received FDA approval, the first robust study of its efficacy was published. This study is referred to as the SAMMPRIS study. (SAMMPRIS stands for "stenting and aggressive medical management for preventing recurrent stroke in intracranial stenosis"—not one of the more elegant acronyms.) In the study, a group of patients similar to Anita was randomized to treatment with all of the medicines we mentioned above or to treatment with these medications and insertion of a stent. Three years after the trial began, an independent review committee stopped it because one group of patients was doing much worse than the other. Unfortunately, the group that had received the stents was having more strokes.

After an average follow-up of one year, 20 percent of the patients in the stent group had strokes, compared with only 12 percent of those in the medicine-only group. That is an increased absolute risk of 8 percentage points, or, in news-report language, a 64 percent increase in the rate of stroke. For every 13 patients who got a stent, 1 of them had a stroke because of the stent alone. Stenting intracranial arteries is a failure and a perfect example of reversal. A procedure that was accepted and deployed was overturned by solid data.

Anita Kramer is disabled, and her stent may be to blame. For one patient, we can never tease apart the gossamer strands of causality (we get into this more in chapter 10), but on average, for patients like Anita, we know it is true. Many were harmed by the stenting.

THE FIRST HARM

Step back for a minute, and consider the case of intracranial stenting. A major, costly intervention for stroke prevention, which was done for a decade and paid for by many insurers, actually increased the risk of stroke.* Moreover, the cost of the therapy was not just the stents. There were the payments to the doctors who placed them. There was also the cost of the brain MRI scans, often done just to look for narrowed arteries in the brain. The only reason these scans were done was to find these stenoses, so some patients could get stents, which did not work. We cannot say how much all this cost, but it was not cheap.

The SAMMPRIS finding exemplifies the first harm of medical reversal. The patients who received the treatment during the years it was in favor were harmed. Anita may be worse off because of the treatment she received. In cases where the treatments did not do harm but simply did not work, patients wasted their valuable time and money. Remember vertebroplasty, the injection of medical cement into fractured bone? A few patients were

---

* Giving credit where credit is due, we should point out that Medicare's stance toward intracranial stenting was a prudent one. Medicare only funded the procedure in the context of clinical research testing its efficacy.

hurt by this procedure, but most simply had their time and money wasted. And it was not just patients' money that was wasted—through Medicare, Medicaid, and other insurances, we all had to pay. The first harm of medical reversal is harm to the patients who undergo the therapy when it is popular and to everyone who has to pay for it.

THE SECOND HARM

The second harm is even more troublesome. One would think that a major study like SAMMPRIS, one that is well done and published in the *New England Journal of Medicine,* would immediately put a halt to the practice. Medical practices, however, are like freight trains—they do not stop quickly. Let us take a look at some of the responses to the article that overturned intracranial stenting. First from Stryker, the maker of the stents, in an article from *USA Today:* "Stryker continues to support the Wingspan Stent System as an FDA-approved Humanitarian Use Device for improving cerebral artery lumen diameter in patients with intracranial atherosclerotic disease who have failed medical therapy." Comments like this, after a well-done, negative study, are hard to understand. Making medical devices is not like being at the helm of a ship. If it sinks, the captain does not have to stay on board. (Maybe the metaphor makes more sense if the ship is full of gold, and the captain cannot bear to part with it.)

If the makers were unwilling to abandon ship because they believed that the treatment still held promise for another indication, their response could have been, "Well, it is back to the drawing board." They could have commenced a randomized trial of the device for another use, perhaps treatment of a subset of strokes in a subset of patients. In this manner, the SAMMPRIS study might have marked the start of a successful therapy rather than the end of a flawed one.

One might question whether one negative study is enough to overturn a practice. If the data that exist in support of the therapy are not strong, and the trial that overturns it is, one study should be enough. (We delve much deeper into what makes data strong and weak in the coming chapters.)

It was not just the device's maker who stood by the product. One of the study's authors noted, "There may be a place for stenting in patients who don't respond well to medical therapy alone." And another prominent researcher noted, "The findings will likely greatly reduce the number of these procedures." There may be a place? Greatly reduce?

This is the second harm of reversal. The contradicted practice does not stop immediately. It continues for years to come. Future patients continue to be harmed by the practice. Although it is terrible that the therapy we gave to Anita might have caused harm, it would be even worse if a similar patient is treated the same way and has the same outcome one year after SAMMPRIS.

We see this pattern, a refusal to abandon a practice that does not work, repeatedly. People with stable angina continue to receive coronary stents years after the practice was overturned by the COURAGE trial (discussed in chapter 1). It is like telling a child not to play with matches, turning around for two seconds, and hearing a match being struck.

Bias in the interpretation of the results of medical trials may play a role here. In a clever follow-up study to COURAGE, researchers reviewed all of the articles that cited the COURAGE trial. Some of those articles agreed with COURAGE, while others argued against the conclusion that stents are no better than traditional medical therapy. Not surprisingly, the articles that took issue with the conclusions were more likely to have been penned by interventional cardiologists (the doctors who place the stents) than were those that were supportive of the findings.

In the case of vertebroplasty, another procedure that we discussed in chapter 1, one doctor wrote, in an accompanying editorial, "When best evidence suggests a toss-up between treatment options and no benefit, informed patient choice is essential." Toss-up? When a treatment is no better than a sham or placebo procedure, that is not a toss-up—that is a failure. We should not offer patients a failed therapy. That therapy should be abandoned.

The same group of researchers who studied the articles about COURAGE also analyzed the medical literature to discover just how long it takes the medical community to abandon a practice after a therapy is proven ineffective. They tracked citations to three major practices that were found not to work: beta-carotene to prevent cancer; estrogen to prevent Alzheimer's disease; and vitamin E to lower cardiovascular risk. They found that 10 years passed before the research community stopped referencing the flawed practice. This estimate of a decade of inertia fits with our own experience. It takes that long for the train of medical practice to stop.

Recently, two physicians published a piece in which they suggested other biases that may play a role in medicine's slow pace of "de-adopting" practices shown not to work. They discussed optimism bias, by which people are more willing to accept and act on information that is in their favor. This bias is certainly magnified when "in their favor" includes monetary benefits. Confirmation bias, the tendency for people to more readily accept information that confirms their beliefs, is almost certainly also at work. Loss aversion is another bias with which we are all familiar. This is the bias that makes casinos profitable. In casinos, people will continue to play because they feel strongly about money that they lost and want to win it back. They are less attached to new winnings (a fact magnified by the presence of chips rather than cash). In medicine, the loss of a trusted therapy is hard to accept. These biases, combined with the strong economic interests often at work, produce the second harm of reversal.

THE THIRD HARM

The third harm of reversal may be the most damaging: the loss of trust in the medical system. There are rare people who think that everything doctors do is either worthless or harmful. These folks are quick to cite any evidence that says some medical practice does not work as evidence for their worldview. We cannot condone this view, but we must acknowledge that medical reversal gives such people something to complain about—even if the conclusions they draw are mistaken.

Although in this book we argue that some medical practices are without value, we know that many others are, without a doubt, beneficial. Our professional lives are spent recommending these therapies. Most people, being both reasonable and intelligent, can be confused by all the flip-flopping in medicine. How can you predict which practices will end up like statins for heart attacks and which will end up like statins for heart failure? In this case, there are two different reasons to take the same pill. The former is beneficial, the latter an example of medical reversal. People should not need to complete medical school in order to make informed decisions regarding their own care. (As we discuss later, the average doctor, who did complete medical school, is still woefully undertrained to think about evidence.)

After the reversal of long-standing mammography screening guidelines, we saw anger directed at the medical community. Fox News published a letter from the head of a breast cancer organization with the headline "Lives Will Be Lost with Proposed Changes to Mammography Guidelines."

Journalists frequently tried to connect this reversal to the Affordable Care Act and interpreted the change as a cost-saving initiative.

Even Jerome Groopman, a thought leader in medical decision making, was irritated by changes in mammogram (and prostate screening) guidelines. In the *New England Journal of Medicine,* he and Pamela Hartzband wrote, "It is neither ignorant nor irrational to question the wisdom of expert recommendations that are sweeping and generic." These authors went on to question whether the task force that changed the guidelines considered the balance between the risk of death and issues important to the quality of life.

We include these arguments here not to question their validity—they are important concerns—but to point out how reversal undermines trust in medicine and makes people just plain angry. Patients are not the only ones who are frustrated; so are their doctors and leaders in the field.

There is another type of harm associated with reversal that we have not mentioned because it is more debatable. This harm occurs when therapies known to offer benefit are withheld because of unfounded concerns about their potential to cause injury. When research shows that such an intervention was safe all along, we learn that we could have been treating patients more effectively all along. Calling this a reversal is a bit of a stretch. Here we are not dealing with an ineffective or dangerous therapy being offered without proof of its benefit, but a beneficial therapy being mistakenly withheld because of concern for its safety. Future physicians learn on their first day of medical school that their first responsibility is to do no harm. Withholding a therapy, when one has doubts about its safety, is generally good medicine. One cannot blame a physician who waits until he is sure not only that the therapy is beneficial but also that it is safe.

This issue is even more complicated because there is a spectrum of how likely the beneficial therapy is to cause harm and of how severe the harm may be. As doctors, we are usually at our most cautious with pregnant women. The thought of doing harm to an unborn child is anathema. It is also not without precedent. Whether from the use of lithium, thalidomide, or diethylstilbestrol during pregnancy, medicine has a long, sad history of using medications, for the supposed good of the mother, that turn out to cause lifelong injury to the child. Withholding treatments, even those known to offer clear benefit to the mother, until they are proved indisputably to be safe is hard to question. On the other hand, withholding treatments based on tenuous physiological arguments, from patients who would likely benefit from them, is more debatable.

In the past 10 years, studies have been done that have overturned long-standing concerns that vaccinations could precipitate flares of multiple sclerosis and that oral contraceptives could precipitate flares of lupus. Another study reversed the practice of delaying spinal anesthesia until a pregnant woman's cervix was dilated beyond 4 centimeters because of the mistaken belief that this would increase rates of cesarean section. Are these examples of good, cautious medicine, where we waited for all the data to be in before offering a therapy? Or are these examples of a unique type of reversal, where proven therapies are withheld for unfounded reasons leading to patients being harmed when they did not receive the best available treatments? This is a tough question, one we do not answer. Instead, we focus on the much more common scenario in which doctors push a therapy for years, only to discover it did not work.

The harms of reversal are threefold. When a therapy is widely deployed before it is proved to work, patients are put at risk. If the therapy turns out to be useless, or even harmful, the patients who received the therapy suffer. The harm may be physical, financial, or both. After the therapy is proved ineffective, further harm continues to be done as the therapy remains in use, supported either unwittingly or by those with vested interests—whether intellectual or financial. Lastly, reversal undermines the trust the public and doctors place in the medical system, and rightly so. In cases of medical reversal, we have put our faith in medical science even though there was no good science to put our faith in. Some extremists use medical reversal to throw the baby out with the bathwater—give up on all of traditional medicine. This is surely a mistake, but, at the same time, it is a consequence of our record of getting some major things wrong.

9
A PRIMER ON EVIDENCE-BASED MEDICINE
:: WHAT IS EVIDENCE IN MEDICINE?

FOR MOST OF US, THE WORD *evidence* evokes scenes of our favorite cop show. Being old-school, we will go with *Law and Order*. "What evidence is there that the defendant committed the crime?" Sam Waterston would ask in a tone implying . . . plenty. Sometimes evidence is definitive: an eyewitness, the defendant's DNA, a motive, a history of violence, and a confession. Usually, however, there are only bits of evidence, but a decision has to be made: Is the defendant guilty? It is seldom easy.

In medicine there are similarly difficult issues. Hypotheses are put forward, a study is done, and then a claim is made. But what is the evidence that this claim is true? Living at high latitudes increases the risk of multiple sclerosis (MS). Women who have twins have more postpartum depression than women who have single pregnancies. These are interesting findings. When these stories come on NPR, we put down our cups of coffee, shush the kids, and listen. Many scientists conduct research on these sorts of hypotheses. The truth is, though, that they interest us, as doctors, only peripherally.

You see, we are clinicians, the kind of doctor who cares for people, the kind you go to when you are sick (or when you are well and want to avoid getting sick). And being a clinician is about one thing, doing something (or knowing when to not do something): making a diagnosis (gallstones); prescribing a pill (atorvastatin); providing a prognosis (your knee injury will get better); performing a procedure (an appendectomy). Doctors have to make decisions about medical practices, the things we do for people. For the claims about MS and postpartum depression, a clinician would pose different, but related, questions. The clinician is not terribly interested in the claim that living at high latitudes causes MS but is very interested in whether taking trips to lower latitudes or adding vitamin D to the diet could decrease rates of MS. The clinician may find the question about the relationship between twins and depression intriguing, but what she really wants to know is, Should she screen for depression in mothers of twins?

Many people think the answers to the scientists' questions and the clinicians' questions go hand in hand. People assume that doing something about the risk for a disease will change the outcome. The truth is, the answers to the scientists' questions and the answers to the clinicians' questions have very little to do with each other. Sure, risk has to exist for clinicians to even pose their questions. No one would think about moving northerners south if there is no risk associated with living in the north, but typically the risk exists no matter what. All of us have some risk of developing MS or depression. Are Swedes at such a high risk for MS that we should treat them differently? The important question here, and this is really key, is whether doing something different changes the outcome. Does screening for postpartum depression really help people feel better?

In medicine, the evidence we need to support a claim depends entirely on the type of claim being made. In the early chapters of this book we present many examples of medical practices that do not produce the desired and expected outcomes. High blood pressure is bad. It increases the risk of death. Atenolol lowers blood pressure, but it does not lower the risk of death. The evidence supporting the claim that hypertension increases your risk of death is very different from the evidence proving that using atenolol to decrease your blood pressure lowers your risk of death. Most studies you read about in the newspaper or hear about on TV and radio are about the former type of evidence. The studies in which you are most interested are about the latter type of evidence.

Perhaps now you are coming to see things from the clinician's perspective. In science and medicine there is nearly an infinite number of interesting questions. In clinical medicine, the only relevant question is: Does this medical practice improve my patient's survival, health, or quality of life? If the answer is no, there is no reason to prescribe this therapy. If the answer is yes, follow-up is warranted: What are the side effects or harms of the treatment? Is the cost of the practice worth the gain?* With all this in mind, let's turn to real claims and see what types of medical evidence are used to support them. This information is critical to understanding what makes evidence strong and what makes evidence weak and to understanding the causes of many of the reversals we experience in medicine.

THE RANDOMIZED CONTROLLED TRIAL

Let's start with a famous claim: simvastatin (a cholesterol-lowering medication) will help someone live longer if the person has high cholesterol and has had a heart attack. This claim was addressed with a randomized controlled trial (RCT), the 4S trial. "4S" stands for the Scandinavian Simvastatin Survival Study. The randomized controlled trial is the gold standard for evidence in clinical medicine. We have referenced these trials continuously in this book as proof of what works and what does not. Randomized controlled trials are experiments. Not the kind of experiments we all performed in high school chemistry and biology. Instead of test tubes and Petri dishes, they involve people.

Until this study was published in the British journal *Lancet* in 1994, simvastatin's effectiveness was not clear. Although high cholesterol was long known to be a predictor of heart attacks, previous attempts to decrease cardiac events by lowering cholesterol had been unsuccessful. Earlier medications had successfully lowered cholesterol, but any reduction in the death rate from cardiovascular causes was offset by increased death rates from other causes.

Like any RCT, the 4S trial was designed in three steps. First, selection criteria were defined, and only people that met these criteria were entered into the trial. In this case, people had to have angina or a history of a heart attack. They also had to have high cholesterol. Second, an intervention is made. In the 4S trial the intervention was the use of either simvastatin or a perfectly matched placebo pill. This is the randomized and controlled

---

* This issue gets complicated when you ask, The cost to whom? To the patient? To the insurer? To Medicare?

part of the randomized controlled trial. Randomization assures that the people in each group are the same, on average. Those participants in the treatment group are no more healthy, wealthy, or wise than those in the placebo group. The control is something as close as possible to the actual intervention but without the active ingredient. Lastly, an end point was chosen. The end point in the 4S study was the ultimate end point, death. The final analysis of the study was a comparison between the number of people who died taking the placebo pill and the number who died taking simvastatin.

The results of the 4S study nicely show how scientists report the results of RCTs. Of the patients in the simvastatin group, 8 percent died, compared to 12 percent in the placebo group. This was an absolute risk reduction of 4 percent. More commonly, researchers report this type of result as a relative risk, the ratio between these numbers, or a relative risk reduction, the percentage decrease in risk because of the intervention. The relative risk in the 4S study was 0.66, and the relative risk reduction was 33 percent. A final useful number is "the number needed to treat" (NNT), the number of patients who must be treated to save one life. In the 4S trial the number needed to treat was 25. (The NNT is the inverse of the absolute risk reduction.) A relative risk reduction always sounds more impressive than a number needed to treat. NPR and *Science Times* usually report relative risk reductions and rarely mention the NNT. In practice, however, the number needed to treat is the more important result. Twenty-five is an impressively low number.

The strength of an RCT is that it is a prospectively planned experiment. The study's design controls for all the factors, other than the planned intervention, that might lead to different outcomes. This is terrifically powerful. Not only are known risk factors for the outcome, such as smoking status, controlled for, but so are those not yet known. Back in 1994 nobody suspected that increased levels of blood vessel inflammation would predict death, but even so, we can be sure that there were approximately equal numbers of "inflamed" patients in each group.

RCTs are not perfect. First, they are expensive studies to perform and require that people agree to be placed in either a treatment or a placebo group. Second, there are subtle ways that RCTs can reach misleading conclusions. We have discussed one situation in which this might happen, when we considered surrogate end points, and we discuss a few more in chapter 10. Lastly, the results of a single RCT do not provide a sort of biblical truth. What they do is present strong evidence about a finding; evidence that often becomes more nuanced as later RCTs examine the same question.

THE COHORT TRIAL

In contrast to the designed experiments that are RCTs, another type of medical study, the cohort study, describes natural, unplanned events. In a cohort study, two groups (cohorts), which differ in some important or interesting way, are identified. These two groups are then followed to discover what proportion of each cohort reaches some predetermined end point. Although the data that come from cohort studies are very similar to those that come from RCTs (relative risk, relative risk reduction, and number needed to treat) there are enormous differences between the two types of studies. While the RCT is an experimental study, the cohort study is an observational study—we do not do anything; we just watch. This difference explains how different study designs can reach different conclusions.

Here is a question: should women take estrogen and progesterone after menopause to lower their rate of heart disease? But first—Why even ask this question? This is where the scientist comes in. We know that during the years when women naturally produce estrogen, they have much lower rates of heart disease than men. After menopause, when their level of estrogen drops, their rate of heart disease rises. Could we maintain women's low rate of heart disease if we gave them estrogen? Time for the clinician to step in. The Nurses' Health Study (NHS), a cohort study begun in 1976, sought to answer this question.

For the NHS, 127,000 nurses, between ages 30 and 55, filled out detailed questionnaires every two years. These questionnaires cataloged medical histories, daily diet habits, and major life events. About 90 percent of the questionnaires were returned, and the data filled more than 600,000 typed pages. With an enormous resource like this, it would seem easy to answer the question. Just make two piles: all the women who took hormones in one pile and all the women who did not in the other. Then see which group did better. More or less, this is what researchers did, and in 1996 they released one of the most cited articles in biomedicine.

According to the NHS, estrogen users had 40 percent fewer heart attacks than women who did not take hormones. A few years later, the NHS confirmed this in women who took estrogen and progesterone compared to women who took neither. Hormones seemed to reduce cardiovascular risk, and with this information in hand, doctors wrote millions of prescriptions.

Of course, you already know what happened, and you probably already know why. The NHS supported the claim that postmenopausal women who take estrogen do better than those who do not. The authors, doctors, and the public took this claim and restated it this way: if a postmenopausal woman starts estrogen, she will do better. Was this claim true?

In contrast to the NHS, the Women's Health Initiative (WHI) was a randomized controlled trial that studied the same topic. A group of women who were past menopause were randomly assigned to hormones or matching placebo pills. It is worth mentioning here an issue about placebos. Many people think that patients in the placebo group get a raw deal. They take a pill that is inert and are lied to about what it is. But the truth is, a randomized trial can only be done, ethically, if there is real uncertainty as to which is better, the treatment or the placebo. In an RCT, both groups are potentially getting the inferior treatment. Having two groups allows the researchers to blow the whistle when one group starts doing worse than the other. Each group needs the other for its protection. The WHI is a great example of a trial in which the placebo group actually did better than those taking the active medicine and, in effect, bailed out the women on treatment.

The Women's Health Initiative randomized 16,000 women, between ages 50 and 79, to estrogen and progesterone or placebo. The women were watched carefully for numerous medical conditions. The study was stopped three years earlier than originally planned, because the women receiving hormone replacement therapy were developing breast cancer, heart disease, stroke, and pulmonary embolism at a higher rate than those receiving placebo. The authors calculated that for 10,000 women over the course of one year, there would be 7 more cardiac events, 8 more strokes, 8 more pulmonary embolisms, and 8 more invasive breast cancers in those receiving hormones compared with those taking a placebo.

The WHI is a landmark study, not just because of its implications for hormone replacement. The WHI implies that even a well-designed observational (cohort) trial can be completely off the mark.

Why did the NHS fail? It is a question that many thoughtful people tried to tackle in the aftermath of the WHI. The bottom line is that the women who took hormones were different from the women who did not. Compared with nonusers, women who used hormones in the NHS were less likely to have a family history of heart disease, be hypertensive, have diabetes, or smoke. They were more likely to take aspirin, birth control pills, and vitamins. They were younger, drank more alcohol, and consumed more saturated fat. They were also wealthier. Researchers call each of these differences "confounders," which are differences between the groups that could be an alternative explanation of the outcome. Maybe it was not the difference in hormone use that caused the outcome; maybe it was one (or many) of the confounding variables.

The authors of the NHS knew what they were doing. They considered confounders. In the 1996 paper they wrote: "Women who take hormones are a self-selected group and usually have healthier lifestyles with fewer risk factors than women who do not take hormones. In general-population samples, hormone users, as compared with nonusers, have more years of education, are leaner, drink more alcohol, and participate in sports more often, even before starting to use hormones."

They then used explanations and statistical adjustments to explain away the effect of these confounders. In other words, the authors seem to say, "Sure, confounders exist, but we anticipated them and adjusted for them and we can still say that hormone replacement reduces heart disease." Reading the NHS today is difficult for us—passages have become classic examples of "eating your words" in the medical literature.

Although it is only a method—like a technique to poach eggs—the randomized controlled trial is best thought of as a medical technology. First devised in the late 1940s (in a study of tuberculosis treatments), the RCT is arguably the most important medical technology of the 20th century. When large and well designed, it is the most powerful way to elucidate the truth in all of medical science. And though it cannot tell you about the mechanism of how a treatment works biologically, it can show conclusively whether a given intervention accomplishes a given goal. In medicine, it is the gold standard for proving a claim.

Observational studies are also useful. They are great at describing the course of medical disease. If you are interested in the rate of lung cancer in nonsmokers, smokers, and former smokers, there is a wonderful cohort study from Denmark that has followed these groups.* Observational studies are also useful for laying the groundwork for an RCT. Observational studies may support a claim that a risk exists or that use of a medication is associated with a better outcome. An RCT can then be designed to investigate whether lessening the risk or using the medication helps people. But when it comes to addressing questions of medical practice, observational studies are sometimes wrong. Notice, we say sometimes. They are not always wrong. If they were always wrong, it would be easy—always do the opposite. Research says observational studies are wrong somewhere between 15 and 50 percent of the time. Unfortunately, we have no way of telling when they are wrong.

CASE-CONTROL STUDIES

There is one more study type we should discuss. Here is a question you might ask: "Does my energy drink increase my chance of getting pancreatic cancer?" Let's begin by noticing how different this question is from the questions we have already talked about. Here, we are asking about something that people already do and whether it is associated with a rare harm.

For several reasons, you cannot do an RCT to answer this question. First of all, RCTs are done to test interventions with potential benefits. You could randomize Red Bull drinkers to a stop-drinking-energy-drinks campaign and then measure pancreatic cancer, but you cannot do the opposite (ask them to drink) if you think the exposure is bad. But more to the point, without some other evidence of harm, launching a "Quit Red Bull" campaign seems unfounded. You need to establish that the hypothesis is plausible. A cohort study would seem an obvious way to answer the question. You could recruit energy-drink users and nonusers, follow them, and compare the outcomes. The problem here is that pancreatic cancer is quite rare, so you would need to enroll hundreds of thousands of people and follow them for years. Such a study would be prohibitively expensive. Who will pay for it? Certainly not the makers of the energy drinks.

Such a situation is where a case-control study becomes useful. Case-control studies generally examine a harmful exposure that potentially

---

* Countries with nationalized health care frequently produce very successful cohort studies. It has been said that every time someone sneezes in Sweden, someone writes it down.

causes a rare event. The studies are retrospective in nature. The researchers start by identifying people who have had the rare event (the cases) and similar people who have not (the controls). The study then looks back in time to discover if the cases were more likely to be exposed to something than the controls. It is like a cohort study run in reverse, starting with the outcome and looking back to the exposure.

These studies can, however, be rife with problems. The cases and controls may differ in regard to things other than the outcome of interest, so the studies tend to run into the same problems with confounders that the Nurses' Health Study did. There also needs to be a reliable way of determining exposure. Can we trust the 60-year-old with pancreatic cancer to accurately recall how many energy drinks he drank in his thirties?

An excellent example of a case-control trial was published in 2000, addressing the concern that caffeine intake causes miscarriage. This question could not be studied in any other way. You could not jump into a costly "stop drinking coffee" RCT, because no one had established that there is any risk to our favorite morning beverage. A cohort study would be difficult because miscarriage is, fortunately, quite rare, so the number of women who would need to be followed would be huge. A case-control study was designed in which women who had miscarried were recruited and interviewed about their caffeine intake. Their use of caffeine was compared with that of women who had successfully carried their babies to term. As in a cohort study, statistical adjustment was required because the patients who had miscarried were different from those who did not: they were older, had had more previous miscarriages, and had less morning sickness. In the end this study showed that women who ingested large amounts of caffeine were about twice as likely to miscarry as those who consumed only small amounts.

Case-control studies, like cohort studies, are not experimental. They are observational studies that cannot prove cause and effect. We do not know that drinking more caffeine puts women at higher risk for miscarriage. We only know that women who ingest more caffeine are more likely to miscarry. It might be the caffeine, or it might be the aggravation caused by their local Starbucks' barista. That said, case-control trials have given us crucial information. These studies have suggested that cigarettes cause lung cancer, that thalidomide causes birth defects, and that people with sleep apnea are more likely to have automobile accidents.

What have we learned? The key to evidence in medicine is the claim. And the most important claim is that some medical practice is beneficial. If you really want to know, you have to do a randomized controlled trial. RCTs are not perfect, but when large and well done, they provide stronger evidence than any other study design. This is a fact that has been well accepted in medicine for at least the past 40 years. Observational studies are useful, particularly for showing the natural history of something: what percentage of heavy smokers will get lung cancer? what percentage of people with hypertension will have a stroke? And case-control studies are great to show whether exposures or habits (often unrelated to medicine) are associated with bad, but rare, outcomes. You can think of each of these studies as the right tool for a specific job. For this analogy, think of the RCT as the hammer, the observational study as the wrench, and the case-control trial as the screwdriver. As it turns out, the clinician is mostly in the hammering business.

10

WHAT REALLY MADE YOU BETTER

:: WHEN EVIDENCE GETS COMPLICATED

IMAGINE YOU ARE WALKING HOME from work and feel your phone vibrate. You pull the phone from your pocket and see that you have a new e-mail. You think, "I'll read it later, but let me just see who it is from." You then notice the subject: "Urgent," and the sender, your boss. You start reading it and the content stops you in your tracks. Suddenly, someone grabs you by the shoulder and pulls you sharply backward. You fall onto the sidewalk. A bus and a rush of hot, diesel-tinged air blows by. On the ground next to you is the stranger who grabbed you. "That guy just saved your life," exclaims an onlooker.

Some of us have had an experience like this during our lives. In a moment, what might have been a life-altering (or life-shortening) event is changed by the action of another person. Without a doubt, the person saved your life. Had that man or woman not grabbed you and pulled, the outcome was clear.

In our world it is easy to talk about cause and effect. Your child is running in the house, bumps the table, and the glass of water sitting on the table spills. "What did I tell you about running?" you say for the twelfth time. The cause (child running) and the effect (water spilling) are clearly linked. Without the former, there would not be the latter. This is how we see the world. Our minds simplify actions and reactions to this sort of cause-and-effect relationship. Often, however, it is not so clear.

Another morning, you are running late to work. Just as you get to your car, you realize you forgot your briefcase (or your keys, or your phone, or your wallet). You run back in to get it and are now five minutes later. As you drive to work, you see a terrible three-car accident. Steam hisses from an engine. People stand around looking shaken. It clearly just happened—maybe five minutes ago. Had it not been for the briefcase, would that have been you?

We begin this chapter with stories of cause and effect to get you thinking about when these relationships are clear and when they are not. In many fields, think foreign policy or finance, it is almost impossible to tease out what would have happened because of the presence or absence of some action. Of course, this complexity does not stop experts from making definitive proclamations. Every day you hear that the stock market went up (or down) because of some report or event. If the relationship were really that predictable, would anybody lose money in the market?

In medicine, it turns out that cause-and-effect relationships are extraordinarily difficult to sort out, probably because the effects of most of our interventions are almost always subtle and complex. For this reason, we argue that only randomized trials can sort out relationships. Among medical studies, only RCTs are experiments, experiments in which you compare identical groups, varying only a single factor, that can delineate whether your intervention has made a difference. But you do not need a randomized trial to determine whether pulling someone out of the way of an oncoming bus is beneficial—it is. However, you do need a randomized trial to determine whether requiring hospital workers to wear gowns and gloves decreases the rate of multidrug-resistant bacterial infections, because there are so many factors contributing to the occurrence of such infections.

This position regarding the necessity of RCTs may seem overly dogmatic. Critics of our position love to cite a tongue-and-cheek article published in the British Medical Journal in 2003. In the article, the authors set out to review all randomized controlled trials examining the benefit of parachutes for skydivers facing "gravitational challenge." Not surprisingly, they found no such trials. The authors noted that free fall is not universally fatal, since some cases of survival have actually been reported. Thus they concluded that the evidence was insufficient to draw firm conclusions about the benefits of parachutes. Because of growing pressure to "medicalize" free fall, the authors closed by calling for a randomized, controlled trial. Noting that it might be hard to recruit people for such a trial, they suggested that "those who advocate evidence-based medicine and criticise use of interventions that lack an evidence base will not hesitate to demonstrate their commitment by volunteering for a double blind, randomised, placebo controlled, crossover trial."

This article was both brilliant and funny and could be republished today as a response to this book. It is often cited when critics argue that we do not need randomized trials for every intervention. But jumping from a plane is very different from taking your blood-pressure medication. The use of parachutes when skydiving is more analogous to the Samaritan pulling you out of the path of a moving bus—the benefit is undeniable. Are there analogous situations in medicine? A case in medicine of an obviously beneficial intervention? Perhaps, appendectomy for acute appendicitis?

TREATMENTS THAT SEEM OBVIOUS

Appendicitis is one of those diseases that most of us have had experience with—either personally or through a friend or family member. The appendix is a vestigial structure, a small pouch that comes off the first portion of our large intestine. Appendicitis is inflammation of this structure caused by a bacterial infection. It is a painful condition that, if not treated, can cause a life-threatening infection of the entire abdomen. Since the 1800s the treatment for appendicitis has been prompt surgical removal of the appendix, appendectomy. If there is an infection in a structure you do not need, you should take it out. Appendectomy was believed to be like a parachute. A person who has an appendectomy remembers pain, and often fever, up until the moment the anesthesia is given. When she wakes up, she feels much better. Appendectomy is the most common emergency surgical procedure in the United States. This is one intervention that many claimed would never be tested in a randomized trial. And yet, we now have four randomized trials that compared appendectomy to antibiotics.

These four trials studied more than 900 patients randomized to either antibiotics (with surgery reserved for those who got worse) or surgery. The results showed that using antibiotics to treat appendicitis may be better than taking people right to surgery. More than 60 percent of the patients did fine with antibiotics alone and did not require subsequent surgery. About 35 percent of the patients who started with antibiotics ended up having the appendectomy. The rates of the life-threatening outcomes, those that made us think surgery was the only option, as well as time in the hospital, are comparable between the two groups: surgery first or antibiotics. The authors of a review of this topic concluded that the best initial strategy for acute, run-of-the-mill appendicitis is antibiotics alone.

In one way the story of appendectomies for appendicitis is just one more example of treatments that seem like they should work until they are proved to not work—or in this case, to not work any better than something less expensive and less invasive. But in another way, it has always seemed especially clear that appendectomies were the best treatment. So if appendectomy for appendicitis is not analogous to the parachute for skydivers, then what is? How about interventions whose benefit seems enormous?

TREATMENTS WITH LARGE BENEFITS

If the magnitude of a benefit is really huge, as in the case of parachutes—you are much, much more likely to survive a jump out of a plane with a parachute than without one—then maybe a randomized controlled trial is not necessary. Consider two problems with this supposition. First, interventions with a sizable magnitude of benefit are rare in medicine. Second, just because an intervention seems to confer a large benefit does not mean that it works.

How common in medicine are interventions that yield tremendous benefits? Tiago Pereira, Ralph Horwitz, and John Ioannidis tackled this question in 2012 in their paper entitled "Empirical Evaluation of Very Large Treatment Effects of Medical Interventions." Pereira and colleagues asked a simple question: if you look at medical trials, how many show very large treatment effects? The authors defined a large treatment effect as a fivefold improvement in an outcome (meaning that, for example, if without treatment you had a 10 percent chance of dying, with treatment that risk should fall to less than 2 percent). In their study they looked at the results of more than 228,000 trials. They found that only 9 percent of the trials demonstrated a very large treatment effect. The topics with large effects were less likely to be about mortality and more likely to be about a laboratory value—it is hard to get a large effect for what really matters. The authors then looked at other studies that addressed the same questions as those that demonstrated the very large treatment effect. Strikingly, they found that 90 percent of the time, the large treatment effects got smaller when you looked at the other studies on the same question. This means that results demonstrating the largest magnitude of effect are more likely statistical flukes than truly important findings. Across all the studies, only one intervention had a large effect on mortality: extracorporeal membrane oxygenation (ECMO), a method to oxygenate the blood of newborns who cannot adequately breathe on their own.* In other words: parachutes are uncommon in medicine.

Accepting that treatments with large benefits are rare in medicine today, the next question becomes, Is there ever uncertainty in the effectiveness of treatments that seem to provide large benefits? If someone proposes a treatment, like ECMO, which leads to survival that far exceeds what we have seen historically, should we just accept it, or is there still the potential for uncertainty? The Milwaukee Protocol for the treatment of rabies is a good example here. The teaching in medical school is that rabies, a virus usually transmitted from the bite of an infected animal (bats, raccoons, dogs), is fatal 100 percent of the time. If you contract it, and you do not get the vaccine before you become symptomatic, you will die. Then in 2005, a 15-year-old girl in Milwaukee developed symptomatic rabies. She was treated with an experimental cocktail (now called the Milwaukee Protocol) of anesthetics and antivirals and survived. This treatment potentially offered a benefit of infinite magnitude. One might ask, why study this?

Of course the real story is complicated. First, it became clear that use of the Milwaukee Protocol did not always cure rabies. Some people died despite receiving this treatment. This was not actually surprising—as no one thought that a treatment for rabies would be 100 percent effective. More recently, research has shown that there may be quite a few people who survive rabies even without treatment. One survey of blood samples from a population in the Peruvian Amazon that has significant contact with vampire bats, revealed that 6 of 63 people tested showed evidence of having survived rabies. Maybe the Milwaukee girl survived despite the treatment.

Rabies is so rare (thankfully) that we will probably never have a random-

---

* Some have argued that the ECMO trial should not even have been done, because the outcome was obvious at the outset.

ized controlled trial of the Milwaukee Protocol, but the example expands the argument that parachutes are rare in medicine. Few treatments promise enormous benefits, and even when they do, the cause-and-effect relationship between treatment and benefit, or the balance of risks and benefits, may be complicated.

This present situation, in which few, if any, treatments are of overwhelmingly obvious benefit, has not always existed. It is probably a symptom of our success. Ninety years ago we did not need an RCT to show that penicillin cured infections that did not previously get better, and we did not need an RCT to show that appendectomy was better than bed rest. Now, however, we need RCTs to show that the newest antibiotic is at least as good as our present ones and that our present antibiotics might be as good as that surgery we have relied on for years.

All that said, there have been some modern medical innovations that are so valuable that they really are like parachutes. One example is imatinib (Gleevec), which, almost overnight, revolutionized the treatment of a type of leukemia. Such innovations are exceedingly rare. Some say, Do not worry, more are coming. These people suggest that we are on the cusp of a new era of medical care and that the advances in this era will be so great, and so obvious, that RCTs will no longer be necessary.

PERSONALIZED MEDICINE

The source of this putative advance is genomic, also called personalized, medicine. In genomic medicine, doctors will tailor therapy specifically to our genetic makeup rather than extrapolating results from RCTs to an individual patient. Thus far, however, experience suggests that genomic medicine will not free us from the need for well-done, experimental studies.

A few years ago, research showed that a cancer drug called cetuximab improved outcomes for patients with colorectal cancer. Since then, oncologists have learned that there are actually two types of colorectal cancer patients—a group of people who benefit from cetuximab and a group of people with certain genetic mutations who do not benefit. The latter group not only does not live longer when treated with cetuximab; they are actually harmed by it. With each passing year, we are discovering new mutations that allow us to better sort the two groups.

Our point is not about cetuximab but about medicine in general, including genomic medicine. Even drugs with great benefit, tailored to a specific mutation and proved to work in randomized trials, may not benefit all the patients we treat. We may not currently be able to detect the small subset of patients who are harmed—not knowing what distinguishes them from those who benefit—and, unfortunately, we still may not be able to make these distinctions for another 20 years. You hear a lot about how personalized medicine will sort out this problem, but although genetic understanding will lead to improvements, the problem will still exist. This issue is a limitation of empirical science; it is a problem of subsets. It will always be impossible for a doctor to know if a particular treatment will help any single patient. All we will ever be able to say is that, on average, this treatment will help many of the patients we think it will.

WHEN RCTs COMPLICATE THE EVIDENCE

Most people agree that RCTs are the best way to prove causality in medicine. RCTs, however, are not magical. They do not always explain away all the complexities that exist in evidence. First of all, not all RCTs are created equal; a poorly done RCT may be worse than a lesser trial design done well. Also, in today's world of industry-designed trials, there is certainly bias in how RCTs are run, analyzed, and reported. We talk more about these issues in chapter 12. But even putting aside these points, RCTs sometimes actually complicate evidence. Even when they are done well, by committed, unbiased researchers who are seeking the truth, RCTs (or their combined data presented in meta-analyses) can lead us astray. It is worth considering three specific ways that RCTs may complicate, rather than clarify, cause-and-effect relationships: accepted error rates; premature termination of trials; and meta-analysis.

:: ERROR RATES IN RCTs

When you begin an RCT, you have two identical groups, one to which you will give the treatment of interest and one to which you will give the placebo. At the end of the study, you analyze these populations to see if they remain the same with respect to the outcome of interest. Your study is considered "positive" if the two populations are now different (meaning that your intervention had an effect) or "negative" if the populations remain indistinguishable. For the rest of our discussion, to make this clearly applicable to medical studies, let us say that a positive study shows a benefit and a negative study does not. So where do statistics come in?

Because your study is only looking at a small number of people, not the entire population, your results will not always be correct—sometimes you will find a difference when there really is one, and sometimes you will not find a difference even when it does exist. There are actually four possible outcomes:

:: You might find a benefit/difference when there is one: a true positive result
:: You might find a benefit/difference when there is not one: a false-positive result
:: You might not find a benefit/difference when there is not one: a true negative result
:: You might not find a benefit/difference when there is one: a false-negative result

Statisticians love to show this in a 2×2 table, which is in fact a very clear way of looking at the situation (despite statisticians' usual love of complexity). See table 10.1.

In designing studies—especially in figuring out how many subjects you will need—you need to choose the level of uncertainty that you will accept. A study without uncertainty would include everybody in the world, but given the cost and complexity of that study, researchers have generally agreed on a level of error they are willing to tolerate. Although any misleading result is bad, a false-negative result is the lesser of the evils. In medicine, a false negative means that we fail to identify an intervention that is helpful. This is bad, but it is not as bad as a false-positive result. A false-

TABLE 10.1

		TRUTH	
		Benefit	*No Benefit*
STUDY RESULT	*Benefit*	True Positive	False Positive (5%)
	No Benefit	False Negative (20%)	True Negative

positive result would lead us to adopt a useless treatment. This contradicts our "First, do no harm" commitment. Traditionally, therefore, we set error levels as follows: a standard trial will fail to recognize 20 percent of treatments that are actually beneficial (false negatives) and will mistakenly identify 5 percent of ineffective interventions as being effective (false positives). These percentages are also shown in table 10.1.

Why are we telling you all this? These error rates become critically important when you try to figure out how likely it is that the studies you read are correct. It turns out that the likelihood that the positive study you read is a true positive, as opposed to a false positive, depends on how likely it was in the first place that the intervention you are studying would work. When we test a new intervention in an RCT, the most optimistic we can ever be that the intervention will be beneficial is 50 percent. This is because, ethically, we can only randomize people to a control group if there is true uncertainty that the treatment will help. We call this ethical principle *equipoise*, and it is a foundation of ethical clinical research. Table 10.2 is a 2×2 table representing studies that have a 50 percent likelihood of being positive. For simplicity the table considers 1,000 studies, 500 of which will study a treatment that is truly beneficial and 500 of which will study a treatment that will fail to live up to expectations. Consider first the beneficial treatments (the left column): we will miss identifying 20 percent, or 100, of them because of where we set the false-negative error rate when we designed the study. Now consider the ineffective treatments (the right column): we will mistakenly identify 5 percent, or 25, of them as being effective. So, in the best of all worlds, if you read 425 positive studies,

TABLE 10.2

		TRUTH	
		Benefit (500)	*No Benefit (500)*
STUDY RESULT	*Benefit*	400 True Positives	25 False Positives (5%)
	No Benefit	100 False Negatives (20%)	475 True Negatives

TABLE 10.3

		TRUTH	
		Benefit (100)	*No Benefit (900)*
STUDY RESULT	*Benefit*	80 True Positives	45 False Positives (5%)
	No Benefit	20 False Negatives (20%)	855 True Negatives

400 of them will be true positives and 25 will be false positives. This is a 94 percent accuracy rate for a positive study. Not bad.

The problem is that for most clinical investigations, there is less than a 50 percent chance that the treatment being evaluated is effective. In fact, the studies that get people most excited are the ones in which an intervention that they never thought would work turns out to be effective. Table 10.3 describes the situation when there is only a 10 percent chance that the proposed treatment is beneficial. In this scenario, if there are 125 studies reporting positive outcome, only 80 of them, or 64 percent, are correct. Thus, almost one-third of the treatments that you would adopt would actually be ineffective. These treatments would eventually turn out to be medical reversals. And remember, these are treatments that you would have adopted based on well-done RCTs, the best evidence available.

The situation is actually probably far worse. In 2005 John Ioannidis published a now-famous article entitled, "Why Most Published Research Is False."* In addition to the unavoidable factors above, Ioannidis pointed out other issues that make a positive study even less likely to be true, including bias in how studies are designed (making them more likely to show a positive result), publication bias (positive studies are more likely to be published than negative ones), and other issues that markedly increase the false positive rate among published studies. We discuss some of these issues in more

---

* This article has been downloaded more than a million times, making it the most read article in the *Public Library of Science* (PLOS).

depth in chapter 12. In the end he concluded that the likelihood that any positive study represents a true finding is probably far less than 50 percent and that even the best randomized trial is only true 85 percent of the time.

:: PREMATURE TERMINATION OF TRIALS

Moving on from error rates, the early termination of trials is another factor that can cause even the best RCTs to complicate the process of proving causality. Imagine you and a friend are playing basketball. He tells you that he is a perfect free-throw shooter.

"What do you mean perfect? Like 90 percent?" you ask.

He shakes his head. "100 percent."

"Come on, that's impossible," you say, knowing that the highest single-season free-throw percentage in NBA history was 98 percent.* There is no way your friend is better than that. "Prove it!"

Your friend steps up to the line and shoots—he makes it. He shoots again—he makes it. One more time—he makes it.

"There you have it," he says.

"Are you kidding me? You made three shots?"

"Three out of three is 100 percent," he says, and walks away.

You are not satisfied.

So, what happened? The problem here was early termination. By dumb luck nearly anyone can make three free throws in a row, but that does not make the person José Calderón. The same is true in clinical trials. An intervention can look exceptionally good, especially if there are only a few outcomes, but if you keep collecting data, the real benefit will become clear.

Why are clinical trials terminated early? We consider it to be unethical to continue a trial once we know that the intervention we are testing is clearly superior (or clearly inferior) to the control. It is no longer fair to the people in the control group (or treatment group) who were recruited with the understanding that we did not know which treatment was superior. However, this perceived ethical necessity can impede the quest for truth. One recent analysis looked at 63 clinical questions for which we had hundreds of studies. Of those, 91 studies were terminated early, while 424 matching studies were completed. The researchers found that studies of an intervention that were stopped early claimed larger benefits of the treat-

---

* José Calderón, Toronto Raptors, 2008–2009.

ment than those studies of the same intervention that ran to a preplanned conclusion. On average, for a given clinical question, if a trial was run to its conclusion and found no effect, a study of the same intervention that was stopped early concluded the treatment was associated with a 29 percent benefit. Just like our basketball shooter, a few lucky breaks, early on, can provide a misleading outcome.

:: META-ANALYSIS

If a single, well-done RCT is good, is the combination of multiple RCTs better? A meta-analysis is a study that quantitatively combines multiple RCTs. Meta-analyses are useful in many ways. They summarize the data from multiple RCTs that study a single topic. They are especially useful when multiple small RCTs have been done but no one single study was powerful enough to reach a conclusion. Sometimes combining these studies can reach a clear conclusion. The disadvantage of meta-analyses is that they study studies rather than patients. Researchers must therefore make choices about which studies to include in their analysis and open themselves to biases inherent in the publication process—not every study has an equal chance of being published.

So which is better, a single, well-done RCT or a meta-analysis of the same question? It would seem that, given the great size, in terms of patients, of a meta-analysis and its ability to consider a more diverse group of patients (owing to the fact that it will include multiple, diverse RCTs), a meta-analysis might win out. This issue was first studied in the late 1990s. A group of researchers compared the results of 12 large randomized trials—with more than 1,000 patients in each arm—with 19 meta-analyses that addressed the same topics but were published prior to the large RCTs. They found significant disagreement between the two methods. If the meta-analysis was positive, only 68 percent of the RCTs were also positive; and if the meta-analysis was negative, 67 percent of the RCTs were negative. Nearly one-third of the time, the results of the meta-analysis and the RCTs were at odds.

When a large, well-done RCT reaches one conclusion and a meta-analysis of the same topic comes to a different one, which is right? Individual RCTs can have exaggerated results because of early termination or idiosyncrasies in the population studied. Thus, if just one or two individual trials are positive and the meta-analysis is negative, we tend to have doubts that the treatment is effective. Conversely, if an excellent and large randomized trial is negative but a meta-analysis is positive, we would be concerned that there is bias at play in the meta-analysis, most likely publication bias. Publication bias occurs because small positive RCTs are more likely to be published than small negative ones. Thus, the medical literature as a whole tends to be biased toward positive results, and meta-analyses will reflect this bias. Finally, if several medium-sized randomized trials and a meta-analysis agree that a treatment is beneficial, then that finding is probably really true.

THE BEST THERE IS

Evidence showing cause and effect in medicine is complicated. There probably are few parachutes (or saviors pulling us from the path of a bus) in medicine. Because of this, we need randomized controlled trials—true experiments that, when done well, prove causation and provide near certainty about treatments. But even RCTs are not perfect, and we will never have RCTs to provide evidence for every decision that needs to be made in medicine. In fact, one reversal we do not talk about extensively—the use of recombinant activated protein C in sepsis—gained prominence based on one RCT but was contradicted by another one. That said, we have come a long way in terms of basing our management decisions on science. As of 2015, thousands of medical practices have been rigorously tested, including some that would have seemed unthinkable to test just 20 years ago.

We end this chapter, which is dedicated to promoting the singular power and importance of the RCT, with a sobering thought: as doctors, the best we can hope for is that, on average, we improve the health of our patients. As patients, the best we can hope for is that a therapy we are offered has a reasonable likelihood of helping us. Although these seem like modest goals, they are dictated to us by evidence-based medicine. It is irrational to expect certainty that every intervention will help. Doctors like to think they help every patient they meet, and patients expect certainty when prescribed a treatment. The practice of evidence-based medicine can increase our confidence in medicine—when a treatment has been shown to improve survival for a group of patients in a large, well-done RCT, doctors should recommend it and patients should accept the recommendation. But at the same time, we know that some subset of those patients—a subset that we have no idea how to recognize—will not benefit.

Making the world a better, healthier place, on average, is the best we can hope for. This modest goal is an admirable one. However, when medical reversal occurs, it is not that a subset of patients did not benefit, it is that doctors did not make the people, on average, healthier; and sometimes they made them worse. On the other hand, when a practice is shown to work in a large randomized trial, although not everyone benefits, people do benefit, on average. This is not trivial. In human history, there are few things we have done that we know brought about net good.

PART **3** **THE ORIGINS OF REVERSAL**

11

SCIENTIFIC PROGRESS, REVOLUTION, AND MEDICAL REVERSAL

EVERY MEDICAL SCHOOL INTERVIEW follows the same script. The interviewer, a doctor taking time out from his practice or research, asks some version of "Why do you want to be a doctor?" The applicant, suited and nervous, responds, "I am interested in science and I want to help people." The savviest applicants make this response sound more profound, but the meaning is always the same. And why not? Medicine is a wonderful field because it offers the opportunity to apply science toward an end that is pure and good. Because of the intricate link between basic science and clinical medicine, medical progress depends on the scientific method. The scientific method, however, when used in medicine, can lead us to adopting therapies before their time. When this happens, the stage is set for medical reversal.

Before we consider the scientific method and its relationship to medical reversal, let us quickly orient ourselves. Up to this point we have presented the "what" and the "why" of medical reversal. The "what" has been the many examples of medical reversal. The "why" has been the reasons these faulty therapies were adopted in the first place. Every example really had the same cause: the therapy in question was founded on flawed data.

We began in chapter 1 discussing medical therapies that were overturned because their use was based on inadequate data—observational studies or mechanistic explanations alone. When these treatments were actually assessed in real, experimental trials, it turned out they were ineffective. In chapter 2, when we discussed subjective end points, we showed how poorly designed studies, those that used inappropriate placebos, have also led to reversal. Chapter 3 extended the list of causes as we covered surrogate end points. Here, evidence was based on end points that are, in themselves, unimportant. When we discussed systems initiatives in chapter 5, we added other types of flawed data, those based on historical controls or studies conducted at a single center.

In part 2 we went even further in explaining the "why." We explained why randomized controlled trials provide our best evidence but admitted that not every randomized controlled trial provides trustworthy evidence. Randomized controlled trials have intrinsic error rates and can become biased when they are stopped early. There is also publication bias, which makes positive studies more likely to be published than equally worthy negative ones. All of these factors increase the likelihood that we will adopt ineffective therapies.

In part 3 we will delve a little deeper into the causes of medical reversal. It turns out that faulty data can be pretty interesting. Sometimes inadequate data exist because of the way the scientific method proceeds, and other times we have inadequate data because of malfeasance. Before we get into juicy stories of manipulated data, let us consider how the scientific method itself can predispose us to reversal. Any proper exploration of this point requires a discussion of the scientific method and Thomas Kuhn. Finally, we end this chapter with another historical lesson, one drawn from a sociologist of medicine whose words more than 30 years ago seem prophetic today.

THE SCIENTIFIC METHOD AND SCIENTIFIC REVOLUTIONS

The scientific method is, at its most basic, a way of determining how the world works. We begin with knowledge in which we are confident; we formulate a question about something we do not yet understand; we hypothesize an answer to that question; and then we design an experiment, an opportunity to observe the world in a controlled and structured way, that will tell us whether our hypothesis is true or false. When done well, the scientific method allows us to extend our knowledge. This is the backbone of biomedical research. For example: we know that our cells have proteins that signal them to grow and proliferate; we also know that some types of cancers produce too many of these proteins; we hypothesize that a drug that disrupts these proteins will slow cancer growth; finally, we design an experiment to see whether our drug works—either on cells in a test tube or in actual people.

But science does not march forward in a clean and orderly way, with each experiment getting us closer to profound and all-encompassing truth. Science proceeds in revolutions. This is the provocative thesis of Thomas Kuhn's book *The Structure of Scientific Revolutions*. First published in 1962, Kuhn's book quickly became influential in the field of the philosophy of science. Although his work has fallen in and out of fashion and has received its share of criticism, it is instructive in understanding how the scientific method can predispose us to medical reversal.

In *The Structure of Scientific Revolutions* Kuhn argued that science proceeds in a series of well-accepted worldviews, or what Kuhn called "prevailing paradigms."* Kuhn believed that there were three key periods in any scientific inquiry. First, there is the "pre-paradigmatic period." During this time scientists lack an organizing theory, or story, to unite their observations. Experiments are haphazard, and theories are proposed only to be quickly abandoned. Usually, many competing theories for how things work are entertained at the same time. Over time, however, one theory or a group of related theories begin to gain traction and coalesce into a broader, explanatory model.

Once a paradigm is accepted, we enter a period called "normal science." During normal science, scientists conduct experiments that reinforce the prevailing paradigm. Many people (and we are among them) think that Kuhn was a bit hard on the so-called normal scientists who do the work during this period. Kuhn makes them seem plodding, doing obvious work. In fact, most of the science we encounter daily is normal science, and it is incredibly important. When a research team announces that they have discovered a gene that increases the risk of breast cancer, that is normal science. The findings are published in major scientific journals and may

---

* The word *paradigm* has since become one of the most abused terms in all of science.

improve health care. They are not, however, revolutionary. We already know that one's genes can increase or decrease the person's susceptibility to disease, and it is normal science to apply this logic to a new problem. If the preparadigmatic period is like completing the straight border of a jigsaw puzzle, normal science is filling in the middle.

Sometimes, while normal science is being done, something disturbing happens: unexpected results occur. Kuhn labeled such results anomalies. An anomaly is an observation that does not quite fit the paradigm. Anomalies are not necessarily negative studies—a negative study can be just as likely as a positive one to support a paradigm. An anomaly is a finding that does not make any sense within the prevailing paradigm. Some anomalies can be incorporated into the paradigm, strengthening the overarching model, but sometimes anomalies accumulate and scientists have to take notice. This is the period Kuhn calls "revolutionary science." Revolutionary science happens when anomalies become so plentiful that the entire paradigm reaches crisis and has to be abandoned. Scientific revolutions are infrequent, according to Kuhn, and this is a good thing. For the most part, paradigms make sense, unite our beliefs, and allow us to explore the natural world. Anomalies are rare events, and they only jeopardize a paradigm when the paradigm cannot be adjusted.

SCIENTIFIC REVOLUTIONS IN MEDICINE

The example that Kuhn most famously used, to illustrate his theory of anomalies and revolutionary science, was the transition from a geocentric theory of planetary motion, in which the planets revolve around the earth, to a heliocentric theory, in which the planets revolve around the sun. Kuhn identified the geocentric view, attributed to Ptolemy, as the prevailing paradigm for 1,500 years. The theory was complicated, but it did a reasonable job of explaining the locations of "heavenly objects."

Then in 1543, Copernicus postulated that all planets revolve around the sun. His theory, however, assumed circular orbits, and as such it did not make better predictions than Ptolemy's did. It also ran against the prevailing interpretation of scripture. Johannes Kepler later modified the theory, substituting elliptical orbits, and now the Copernican model made better predictions about where planets should be at any given time.

The anomalies to the Ptolomean paradigm began to accumulate. Most importantly, in 1610, Galileo observed that Venus has phases (like the moon does). This fact could only be reconciled with a heliocentric, and not a geocentric, model of the solar system. This example, though a good one, is a little different from the classic progression that Kuhn describes, in the sense that the new paradigm came a little before the anomalies—it usually is the other way around.

Medicine has seen an occasional revolution, a discovery that completely changes the way we understand health and disease. The introduction of the germ theory of disease was certainly one of those. The prevailing paradigm before germ theory was that (what we now know are infectious) diseases were transmitted by miasma. Miasma, or bad air, came from decomposed matter. A local epidemic, for example, would be blamed on the presence of miasma, since the idea that a disease could be passed from person to person had not yet been conceived.

There have been more recent revolutions in areas of medicine.* Until the 1980s, the prevailing paradigm was that peptic ulcer disease was a disease of overproduction of, or sensitivity to, acid in the gastrointestinal tract. There was clear evidence that certain exposures (extensive skin burns, cigarette smoking) made one more prone to ulcers, and there were treatments (antacids, surgery) that worked to heal the ulcers. However, there were anomalies that upset this paradigm. There were no convincing data that explained why some people got ulcers and others did not. And then there was this bacteria, probably first recognized in the 19th century, that seemed to live in the acidic environment of the stomach. In the 1980s Drs. Barry Marshall and Robin Warren were finally able to isolate the bacteria (*Helicobacter pylori*) and eventually prove its link to peptic ulcer disease.[†] A revolution: a disease that was thought to be caused by acid production alone and treated primarily with antacids now became an infectious disease treated primarily with antibiotics. Even today, though, the peptic-ulcer story remains open. We don't fully understand why, of all the millions of people in the world who are infected with *H. Pylori*, some develop disease but others do not.

Medical research frequently produces anomalies. When we are surprised

---

* Honestly, it is often hard to decide what to call a revolution and what to call an anomaly that has a greater-than-average impact on the prevailing paradigm.

† For this discovery, Drs. Marshall and Warren received the Nobel Prize in Physiology or Medicine in 2005.

by the results of a study, it is often because the results run counter to our worldview. We thought we understood a disease process and based a hypothesis on this understanding. When the hypothesis is disproved, we are forced to reconsider our understanding. Only rarely do anomalies accumulate and culminate in a revolution. More commonly, our understanding of the disease process is tailored to accommodate the new data.

SCIENTIFIC PROGRESS AND MEDICAL REVERSAL

Some medical reversals are anomalies in the Kuhnian sense of the word. Reversal occurs because doctors adopt a therapy based on their understanding of the prevailing paradigm. When that treatment is proved ineffective, it not only is an anomaly, upsetting the paradigm; it also becomes a reversal. Other reversals do not represent anomalies. In these cases, doctors have adopted a therapy that does not really fit with the prevailing paradigm. When this therapy is reversed, it does not raise doubts about the paradigm; instead, it forces doctors to acknowledge that their practice made little sense within the paradigm.

In chapter 1 we discussed the COURAGE trial. COURAGE showed that even though chest tightness (angina) is caused by blockages in the coronary arteries that deprive the heart of oxygen, and even though those blockages can be remedied with stents, those stents do not save lives and offer minimal (if any) subjective benefits. Was this reversal an example of an anomaly, or an example of a result alerting doctors that their therapies were at odds with the paradigm? To answer this question, it is worth first briefly considering the history of the two cardiac processes that stenting addresses: angina and heart attacks (myocardial infarction, or MI).

The first published descriptions of angina appeared in the late 1700s. Some of the most accurate descriptions of this syndrome have been attributed to Dr. William Heberden. At the time, the exact cause was unknown, and treatments were symptomatic—"quiet and warmth, and spirituous liquors," as well as opium. Great strides in the understanding of angina came in the late 19th century, and by the early 20th century, angina had gone from a syndromic description of chest pain to a symptom clearly related to blockages of the coronary arteries—a symptom that carried a poor prognosis.

The 20th century also saw the coalescing of a paradigm concerning the understanding of the MI. Although the first accurate description of the process may date back to 1844, it has only been in the past 25 years that plaque rupture has been accepted as the causative event in most MIs. The idea is that the walls of diseased, atherosclerotic, coronary arteries are unstable. If an atherosclerotic lesion ulcerates, or ruptures, it releases factors that can cause thrombosis, blood clotting, within the vessel. This blockage then leads to the death of heart muscle, the definition of an MI. The process of plaque rupture can occur in narrowed arteries, those that are causing angina, or in the walls of vessels that are diseased but not narrowed to the extent that they would cause symptoms.

Reviewing the current paradigm of angina and MIs informs how the results of the COURAGE trial can be viewed. As far as MIs are concerned, the idea that stenting stable lesions would be preventive made little sense. Plaque rupture can occur in any vessel, not necessarily the ones that are narrowed enough to cause angina. The finding that stenting does not save lives is not an anomaly; it just reinforces that the hypothesis made little sense within the paradigm. (Shockingly, however, a recent study found that 90 percent of patients believed the procedure would extend their lives and 88 percent believed it would prevent a future heart attack.)

For angina, the interpretation is more complicated. Placing stents does improve symptoms—this finding was expected, given the century-old paradigm holding that narrowed vessels cause angina. The fact that the benefit was as small as it was, compared with modern medical therapy, may someday be seen as an anomaly. The sham studies that we propose (chapter 2) would lend clarity to this issue.

HOW SCIENCE AND MEDICAL SCIENCE DIFFER

There is a critical point to make when we apply Kuhn's thinking to medical sciences. Unlike pure science, medicine directly affects the lives of human beings. No one was really hurt when we believed in Ptolemy's astronomy—we do not think anybody got lost on a misdirected space voyage in the third century. When a medical hypothesis turns out to be wrong, there is the potential for injury. Medical paradigms are the theories that help us understand the biology of health and disease. These theories are supported by diverse data—laboratory research, case-control studies, and observational studies. Medical science is a relatively new field that operates on well-developed scientific method; because of this, our paradigms have been robust. Revolutions in the modern medical sciences have been rare and limited, affecting minor paradigms in limited areas of the field. The greatest advances of the past century replaced preparadigmatic thinking and established paradigms.

When medical science functions properly, medical paradigms suggest hypotheses: for example, the hypothesis that tight blood-sugar control benefits diabetics. The next step in the scientific method is to test this hypothesis, in this case by a randomized trial testing whether strict blood-sugar control is better than lenient control. If the hypothesis is proved true, the paradigm is strengthened. If false, the paradigm is adjusted or an anomaly is recorded. Reversals happen when we jump the gun, when doctors start acting based on the paradigm rather than on the experimental results. They act as if the hypothesis is true, and the experiment is performed only years later, if at all.

Anomalies become reversals when we have already implemented them broadly, believing the theory to be the truth. Had people not yet been treated, we could say, "Back to the drawing board; let's think more about that paradigm." Thus, anomalies can be reversals, but they do not have to be. If a medical intervention is thoroughly tested before it is implemented and found to be in error, the theory is adjusted and no one is harmed.* This is the process every time a drug in development fails to make it to the pharmacy. This is the appropriate way to address anomalies. However, an anomaly that becomes a reversal can have a direct and negative effect on a human being who is ill. This does not happen in the nonmedical sciences.

WHY IT IS WORTH THINKING ABOUT KUHN

Before moving on to discuss more concrete causes of reversal, let's consider three more lessons from Thomas Kuhn. First, Kuhn had the wisdom to realize that history books whitewash the missteps. In the modern world, there is better documentation of the past, but medical books still underemphasize how wrong we have been at times. It is hard to believe that just 15 years ago there was nearly universal enthusiasm for hormone-replacement therapy in postmenopausal women. Some practitioners' current embrace of treating age-related testosterone decline in men suggests how completely we have forgotten our error. Because history underemphasizes how fervently smart people believed things that turned out to be wrong, we find it

---

* In the medical literature this is often called translation failure.

hard to believe that things we currently believe might someday be proved wrong as well.

Second, Kuhn saw experiments as tests of our current worldview, the current paradigm. This is how we should look at clinical trials in medicine. Our understanding that narrowed coronary arteries cause angina is supported by countless studies, but the COURAGE trial is an experiment that may have demonstrated an anomaly. In the future, we may reach a better understanding of how pain is caused by narrowed arteries, and this knowledge might suggest a different intervention that saves lives and improves symptoms.

Third, Kuhn reminds us that we have to design experiments that challenge our worldview. We should not only do experiments meant to support the paradigm. Although these experiments are important, they do not offer the potential advances that experiments questioning key assumptions do. This was the foundation of Kuhn's contempt for "normal science." In doing any type of medical science, though, be it normal or paradigm-questioning, you have to wait and see whether the proposed intervention works before you implement it. No theory in the history of science has been ironclad; the only way to know something works is to know it works.

JOHN MCKINLAY

In the final stretches of putting this book together, we came across the work of Dr. John McKinlay, whom we referred to in the introduction. McKinlay is a sociologist of medicine, who, before hormone-replacement therapy and antiarrhythmics for heart attacks, provided an outline for how medical practices come into vogue and fall out of favor; his outline is remarkably similar to our own research and understanding. McKinlay described "seven stages in the career of a medical innovation," and it is worth revisiting those stages, highlighting what has changed and what remains the same.

In 1981 McKinlay suggested that innovations are first announced with a "promising report," often noting success in a patient and published in a prominent medical journal. In the second stage, the profession adopts the innovation, motivated by the belief that the innovation will benefit patients (as well as by some peer pressure and financial incentives). Stage three occurs when patients and payers accept the innovation as standard. In the fourth stage, "data" begin to enter the story. However, the data supporting the innovation come only from insubstantial studies that support the inno-

vation in the most superficial way. In stage five, we see the first randomized controlled trial assessing the intervention. These studies may either
support the innovation or prove that it is ineffective (medical reversal).*
Stages six and seven are the reactions doctors have to the data; first denial,
as entrenched interests deny that the innovation may not be effective and
then, finally, acceptance. McKinlay's conclusion about the solution to the
problem is the same as ours: "All services must be evaluated objectively
(preferably and where appropriate by RCTs) before they are introduced."

So what has changed? Well, first, today a promising report takes many
forms. McKinlay described it as a small pilot study, while today a promising report could be anything from a basic science or anatomical paper, an
observational study, or a randomized trial that uses an inappropriate control
arm, an unimportant end point, inadequate follow-up, or poor blinding. In
fact, with the rise of the influence of the biopharmaceutical industry, more
and more often, promising reports come in what appear to be well-done
randomized trials, whose flaws are revealed only upon careful scrutiny.

Second, the role of perverse financial incentives likely plays a greater role
in health care today than in 1981. In 1981 health-care spending in America
as a percentage of GDP was 8 to 9 percent, while in 2014 that number is 18
to 20 percent. As many have noted, all these dollars have not yielded a pro-
portionate increase in life expectancy, and in that sense the United States
lags behind many other industrialized nations who spend less. These trends
have also changed McKinlay's narrative. Professional organizations and
pharmaceutical companies have a strong interest in more medicine and a
greater reluctance to abandon what has been disproved. In the next chapter
we explore these forces in more depth. For now, we must marvel that John
McKinlay saw so much of what was to come when evidence-based medicine was still in its infancy.

---

* Of course, McKinlay did not use the term medical reversal.

12

SOURCES OF FLAWED DATA

EVEN THE BEST RANDOMIZED controlled trials, or practice guidelines based on such trials, can mislead us. Doctors can read the literature, carefully analyze the trials, adopt only therapies that seem well-founded, and still offer treatments that turn out to be wanting. This is not only because sometimes we discover anomalies or work from incomplete paradigms. It is also because, in today's world of biomedical research, many studies are funded by the pharmaceutical industry. There is a great temptation to create bias when the very companies that develop the drugs, devices, and infusions also design the studies that test whether these products work. How this bias is introduced varies. It may occur within individual studies in which the design is subtly skewed to favor one outcome. It may be present in how the results are promulgated—companies decide how and when to report studies. When companies hold back evidence, the medical literature becomes just the tip of the trial iceberg—a handful of trials, selectively drawn from a much larger pool. Each year we discover new ways that bias has been introduced, new ways that we have been fooled—reasons why trials we believed were accurate were, in fact, not.

There are three key ways doctors are actively misled into practicing medicine that is at high risk of reversal. First, the pharmaceutical and med-ical-device industry can manipulate studies. Second, treatment guidelines, often considered helpful and unbiased by physicians, can endorse treat-ments that are not evidence-based. And, third, the approval process for medical therapies often sets the bar too low.

INDUSTRY-SPONSORED TRIALS

Just days after the story broke, the Internet coined a term for the whole affair: "Scamiflu." In the spring of 2014, a meta-analysis that appeared in the *British Medical Journal* presented data that showed that oseltamivir (Tami-flu), a medication used widely to treat the flu (influenza), provides very little benefit—even less than was previously thought. This drug, which had been on the market for more than a decade, had been studied in the past, but unlike previous studies, this meta-analysis was performed by indepen-dent researchers who had unrestricted access to full study reports of every oseltamivir trial (published and unpublished). Although Tamiflu had been thought to prevent transmission of the flu virus, decrease hospitalizations, and save lives, the study found it did no such thing. Tamiflu decreased flu symptoms by less than a day, from an average of seven days to just over six. It did this while causing nausea and vomiting. The drug did nothing to pre-vent transmission of the virus or reduce hospitalization. Finally, there was no evidence that it decreased deaths.

These findings were particularly unfortunate because countries around the world had stockpiled Tamiflu for years in preparation for a potential epidemic. Between the United States and the United Kingdom, more than $2 billion was spent to amass Tamiflu stockpiles. Government stockpiles were justified because officials believed that the drug could be used to slow the spread of a future influenza epidemic and save lives. It makes no sense to stockpile a drug (at tremendous cost) that is no better than Tylenol. The case of Tamiflu is another example of medical reversal, a therapy adopted into widespread use that is later found to be no better than our previous less expensive and safer therapy. It is a particularly costly, visible, and pain-ful example that deserves deeper analysis because it illustrates ways that industry-sponsored trials can mislead physicians.

Before we can delve into the details of the Tamiflu case, there are some basics you need to know about the flu. First, when people talk about "the flu," most of us are really talking about influenza-like illnesses. You have probably experienced at least one of these—you develop fever, cough, aches, and pain. Among people with influenza-like illnesses, some are actually infected with a virus called influenza, while other patients have been infected with other viruses—rhinovirus, coronavirus, and others. These viruses can cause illnesses that mimic true influenza. There is a test to distinguish influenza from influenza-like illnesses; however, for practical reasons, doctors have traditionally not used this test very often. If the treatment is to go home, eat some soup, take some Tylenol, call in sick to work, and get some sleep—does it matter if you have rhinovirus or influenza?

Influenza can be a terrible infection. It accounts for more than 100,000 hospitalizations each year in the United States and more than 50,000 deaths. In the worst years, the numbers can be terrifying. The 1918 Spanish Flu pandemic killed between 20 and 100 million people. Influenza is especially dangerous for people at the extremes of age and for women who are pregnant. Influenza can kill by filling the lungs with secretions, by damaging the lung tissue, or by causing a massive inflammatory reaction. The patients with severe influenza can also develop secondary infections, most dangerously, bacterial pneumonia.

With these facts in mind, let us turn to Tamiflu. When doctors and policymakers set out to judge this new pill to fight "the flu," they studied patients with influenza-like illness. The appropriate end points they needed to study were hospitalization, pneumonia, transmission of the virus, and death. Most of the trials considered in the 2014 meta-analysis by the *British Medical Journal* group studied these very outcomes in these very patients.

Roche, the company that manufactures Tamiflu, seemingly working to help us make our point that companies can successfully introduce bias into studies, published its own meta-analysis just one month before the BMJ article. The Roche-sponsored study found that Tamiflu had a large benefit, reducing deaths among patients who were later proved to have influenza, especially if they took the drug early in the course of their illness.

Why were Roche's results so different from those of the BMJ authors? Roche's study combined data from observational studies, case-control studies, and randomized trials. It included only people who were proved to have influenza (rather than those with influenza-like illness) and focused on people who received the drug early. These are not unimportant data, but they do not pertain to how the drug is used in the real world.*

To know the real-world utility of Tamiflu, we need to know whether it helps all the people who were told to take it—not just those who later turn out to have true influenza. The question facing doctors is, By giving Tamiflu to all patients that you suspect have "the flu," do you improve outcomes? Simply studying patients who are later confirmed to have influenza—and not all the patients you treat—is misleading. Not to mention that observational data are terribly unreliable for this question. Patients who did not receive Tamiflu (or did not receive it early) were likely very different from those who received the drug early. Even if you considered all the differences you could think of (patients' other medical conditions, socioeconomic status, access to care . . .) and adjusted for them, it is still unlikely that you would have controlled for all the factors that predict worse outcomes for the untreated people.

The problem of industry-sponsored bias is not unique to Tamiflu; it is ubiquitous in research that is paid for by the pharmaceutical industry. We know this because there are other ways to get your research funded, and we can compare research supported by different sorts of funding. Trials are also paid for by agencies that do not have a vested interest in one outcome or another—agencies such as the U.S. National Institutes of Health, the Veterans Administration, and the Department of Defense. Additional funding is obtained through nonprofit grants, private funds, cooperative research groups, and charitable organizations. An investigation published in the BMJ in 2008 compared industry-sponsored trials to trials paid for by other entities. The authors found that industry-sponsored studies were more likely to reach positive conclusions regarding the benefits or cost-effectiveness of a therapy and more likely to test a new therapy against a placebo (as opposed to a real competitor). When considering both original trials and meta-analyses, industry-sponsored studies are four times as likely to reach a positive conclusion.

Two other findings in the comparison of industry- and non-industry-sponsored research warrant note. First, industry-sponsored studies are less

* These data do suggest that as we go forward, tests for influenza should probably be used more regularly.

likely to be published or presented, or to have been published after a delay, than nonindustry research. Second, and perhaps surprisingly, if you score the quality of industry-sponsored studies by any set of trial-design criteria, industry-sponsored research scores just as highly. How can we make sense of these findings?

The first issue gets at selective reporting. Selective reporting happens when only *some* of the trials that get conducted on a question of interest are reported. The trials that we see are preferentially those that were positive. This was part of the reason that an earlier analysis of Tamiflu, published by the same group as in the recent BMJ article, concluded that the drug worked. For that analysis, the investigators only had some of the data, and those data looked good. It is not hard to understand why selective reporting leads to bias in the literature. It is the same reason why letters of recommendation are almost always positive. Anyone can find three people willing to say something nice about them—the breadth of opinion is only revealed by consulting everyone they know.

The second issue, that industry-sponsored studies appear to be as methodologically sound as nonindustry studies, emphasizes the inadequate measures by which we judge the quality of medical research. When we examine a randomized, double-blind, placebo-controlled trial, we see that industry-sponsored researchers do just as well at randomizing and blinding the participants. However, the criteria we use to evaluate the research evaluate just a few, very basic, measures. This is the equivalent of checking to see if a person has a pulse and concluding that he is in good health. It is not surprising that the industry does just as well on these measures—the way in which bias is introduced is subtle (and creative).

Recently, one of us noticed a worrisome discrepancy in a trial comparing two drugs. The trial called for doses of the drugs to be reduced if patients experienced prespecified adverse effects. When the trial started, the two drugs were dosed equivalently, but if a patient required a dose reduction, the dose of the industry drug fell a bit, while the dose of the comparison drug fell a lot. This kind of trial design does not routinely set off any warning bells—the bias in the design is easy to miss—but it shows how hard it is to develop a scale to catch all the small ways a trial may be biased.

Given these points, it should not be surprising that physicians are more wary of industry-sponsored trials than those sponsored by governmental or nonprofit groups—collectively called nonconflicted bodies. Aaron

Kesselheim and colleagues proved this in a recent study. The authors randomly assigned doctors to read summaries of a hypothetical study. Some doctors were told that the pharmaceutical industry funded the study, and others were told the National Institutes of Health (a nonconflicted body) did. The rest of the text was identical. Across the board, physicians were less confident in the results and less likely to support the drug if the trial was funded by industry.

Some use this paper to argue that criticism of industry trials is excessive because doctors are already skeptical of industry trials. Instead, we conclude that Kesselheim's finding is reassuring. Industry sponsorship should set off our "spidey sense," because bias is often detected only in the fine print and introduced in complicated, nuanced, and creative ways. Industry-sponsored trials do a masterful job at meeting the basic requirements for a good trial, and doctors have to look far beyond article summaries to find the reasons to be skeptical. There is another problem with this study, but we will save it for interested readers in the footnote.*

CONFLICTS OF INTEREST IN PRACTICE GUIDELINES

Doctors do not have time to read all the research that is out there. Most of our time is spent caring for patients. For those of us in academics, we are also trying to squeeze in teaching and scholarly activity. Our colleagues say that they can rarely read 10 articles a week, let alone read every paper with the fine-tooth comb needed to pull out every little bit of bias. For this reason, we rely on professional societies and teams of experts to synthesize the data on important medical questions and develop broad treatment principles. This task is almost never easy. Developing a guideline requires sifting through heaps of sometimes-conflicting data, weighing the risks and bene-

---

* The other problem with the study is the use of priming. Priming means that people give you the answer you told them to give. At a simple level, it is the difference between asking, "What color was the car?" versus "The car was white, wasn't it?" In the study by Kesselheim and colleagues, a close look at the methods reveals that three times, prior to the survey, doctors were reminded that the study they were participating in was "not associated with any pharmaceutical manufacturer." This repeated mention of funding source arguably primed readers to be more vigilant about the funding source of research. In a way, Kesselheim and colleagues may have inadvertently sown the seeds for the results of their study in their repeated insistence that it was not industry funded.

fits of treatments, and trying to come to a definitive recommendation. This needs to be done while recognizing that the data you need most might not exist or might not be available. Not surprisingly, guideline groups sometimes reach controversial conclusions.

In 2013 joint guidelines from the American College of Cardiology and the American Heart Association made a controversial recommendation for using cholesterol-lowering statin drugs for primary prevention— treating healthy people to prevent them from having a heart attack or stroke. The group recommended that people who have never had a cardiovascular event (such as heart attack) should take a statin if their ten-year risk of a cardiovascular event is greater than 7.5 percent. Some estimate that if this guideline is widely adopted, the number of Americans taking a statin will increase by 12.8 million people. If followed globally, the ACC/AHA recommendations could result in more than a billion people taking a statin. The ACC/AHA recommendation is an enormous public-health intervention.

Whether the ACC/AHA got it right or wrong is controversial and could be (and probably will be) the topic of a book by itself. What is known for sure is that statins have real benefits and real side effects and that the effects on overall mortality, when statins are taken by healthy people, are uncertain. It is therefore fair to have a debate about the ACC/AHA recommendation and how it was reached. One of the more troubling aspects to consider is that half of the guideline committee panelists had financial ties to the manufacturers of statins. You have to question whether the members of the committee were acting impartially or whether they were influenced by the money they had been paid.

The problem with financial conflicts in guidelines is several-fold. Some guidelines are commissioned by professional societies that receive a large chunk of funding from industry. Drug companies themselves may sponsor guidelines. Eli Lilly provided 90 percent of the funding behind guidelines for septic shock, called "Surviving Sepsis." It surprised no one that Lilly's own drug, Xygris, was recommended prominently. Xygris turned out to be an example of medical reversal when a 2012 randomized trial found no benefit of the drug in sepsis. A guideline may also be tainted when a panelist has received or is receiving payments or royalties from industry. In chapter 15 we discuss other, nonfinancial, ways that guidelines may be tainted, but what is clear is that guidelines are almost certainly influenced by financial conflicts of interest. When a recommendation is made in the setting of these conflicts, groundwork for a future reversal is laid.

THE FDA APPROVAL PROCESS

Another way our medical system predisposes us to medical reversal is a lenient standard for the approval of new therapies. When drugs, devices, and procedures are allowed to come to market without clear evidence that they work (yet are paid for by the government and insurers), conditions are ripe for reversal.

The U.S. Food and Drug Administration gets criticized from all direc tions. Proponents of evidence-based medicine criticize approvals for coming too early, without clear evidence that a drug works. The pharmaceutical industry and patient advocates often fault the FDA for taking too much time to make decisions, thus stifling "progress." Working at the FDA is a hard job. In our experience, FDA regulators are some of the smartest and most sincere people in the business. They are trying to do the best they can, balancing diverse interests and pressures, within the rules mandated by Congress. For example, the FDA cannot consider cost as part of its deliberations, even though the United States does not have a group of experts (as many European nations have) who subsequently balance costs and benefits following a drug's approval. The FDA has a mandate to ensure safety and efficacy, but not comparative efficacy. If a company develops the eighth statin drug, the FDA cannot demand that the company prove that this drug is more effective than the cheaper ones that are already on the market.

Our position here is obvious: because we are concerned with medical reversal, we favor higher standards for approval upfront. Drugs, devices, and procedures should not be debuted unless we have good evidence that they work or unless a trial adequately testing whether they work has recruited all its participants and is ongoing. To emphasize how critical this stance is, we focus on three areas related to the FDA approval process, all of which predispose us to adopt therapies before their time. Two of these issues are directly related to the FDA approval process: the standards for device approval and the process known as accelerated approval. The third issue is a striking example of pharmaceutical-company malfeasance: off-label marketing.

:: DEVICE APPROVAL

Medical devices are a serious matter. These constructs of plastic, metal, and batteries are often implanted within the body. The purpose of a medical device is to ease suffering or prevent death. Common examples are artificial joints and pacemakers. In principle, thinking about a device is no different from thinking about a pill. If a new pill is developed and claims to reduce chronic back pain, it should be tested before we use it. Assemble a group of people in whom you think it might work, randomize them to the pill or placebo, and monitor pain scores. Follow these people for months or (ideally) years, and observe whether the drug has any benefit and whether that benefit persists over time. Chronic back pain is a persistent condition. The classic placebo response would be an initial benefit that gets smaller over time.

Now, let's say that instead of a pill, the treatment at issue is a neurosurgically implanted electrical stimulator. The theory is that the device provides gentle electrical current to nerve roots and reduces pain. How should we test this device? The standard is the same. Assemble people in whom you hope the device will work, randomize half to the device, and the other half to ... Here, it gets complicated. Ideally, you would actually randomize your participants to three groups. One group would get the actual device. One group would have a sham device, an inert box, implanted. The last group would get the best management they could without the implantation of any hardware. If the stimulator's effect is real, only the group with the working device will have a benefit. If the effect is that of a placebo, both the real and the sham device groups will improve. If all groups are identical, then the device does not even have a placebo benefit. If the medical-management group does best, then you have to worry that the device is actually causing pain.

Unfortunately, the logical trial we describe is rarely done. Spinal-cord stimulators really do exist but have been compared only to medical management in small, randomized trials (of about 100 people) or against a surgical operation (itself not proved) in even smaller studies. The stimulators used in clinical practice have never been compared to a sham device. Some stimulators were approved based only on "before and after studies," which showed that a few dozen patients' symptoms improved after receiving the device. This low bar for device approval is especially concerning because most devices have the potential to cause harms. In the case of spinal-cord stimulators, nearly 20 percent of patients experience electric lead migration; in other words, the wires end up somewhere different from where they were placed. There are many other dangerous complications, the risks of which might be worth taking if the stimulator was actually known to work.

For another example of the low standards that are currently the norm for the approval of medical devices, we look to the work of Sanket Dhruva, Lisa Bero, and Rita Redberg, who systematically examined the strength of evidence behind the FDA approval of high-risk cardiovascular devices. In 123 studies supporting the approval of 78 devices, randomized trials accounted for only 27 percent of studies (and remember, we are still not talking about comparison to a sham device). Nearly one-third of studies used historical controls, which, as we have discussed, are notoriously prone to bias. The vast majority of studies (88 percent) had a surrogate end point as the primary one, and 78 percent of studies had discrepancies in the number of patients assigned to a treatment and the number that were subsequently analyzed. As the experience with Tamiflu made clear, you have to consider outcomes in all the patients you assign to treatment, not just in those who are most likely to benefit.

:: ACCELERATED APPROVAL

In the early 1990s, with the experience of the HIV/AIDS epidemic, the FDA pioneered the accelerated-approval program. This program allows drugs for serious diseases, diseases for which there are few treatment options, to gain approval by showing benefit on a surrogate end point that is reasonably likely to predict a clinical benefit. After approval is granted, the drug is given a period of time to prove that it benefits a more important end point. Since the adoption of this program, hundreds of drugs have gained FDA approval in this manner.

Accelerated approval is not a bad idea. The problem is that it has not been instituted as originally designed. Confirmatory studies seldom come quickly. Often, studies have not completed participant enrollment (or have not even begun) when approval is granted. After a drug is approved, it is much harder to get participants to sign up for a study. Too often, confirmatory studies never get completed. In 2009 the Government Accountability Office summarized the experience of nearly 20 years of accelerated approval. Although fully one-third of postapproval confirmatory studies had not been completed, the FDA had never removed an "accelerated-approval" drug from market. This included examples in which companies had been delinquent in providing confirmatory data for as long as 13 years.

In 2010 the FDA finally stood its ground. The agency revoked the approval of bevacizumab for breast cancer. (We talked about bevacizumab in connection with surrogate outcomes in chapter 3.) The drug had initially been shown to slow the growth of breast tumors, but multiple studies failed to replicate this finding, and the drug had absolutely no benefit on survival. The decision to remove the approval for bevacizumab generated an outcry, but it was based on rigorous data analysis. Despite the revoked approval, many insurance companies continue to pay for bevacizumab for the treatment of breast cancer, and the National Comprehensive Cancer Network (NCCN), an alliance of 25 cancer centers, continues to recommend it in its guidelines. Because Medicare must pay for anything recommended by the NCCN, Medicare must pay for the off-label use of a drug that has not been proved to work and which the government's own agency has condemned. The case of bevacizumab shows just how hard it is to take away a drug that was granted accelerated approval.

Accelerated approval needs to operate in the way it was intended. The benefits of the program are obvious—if a drug goes on to make a positive difference, then the more people that get early access to it, the better. But there are potential risks. A drug might turn out to be ineffective, or even harmful. For the system to work, drugs must be subjected to a confirmatory study in a reasonable length of time. If a drug is found to be ineffective, the health-care industry must accept the data and quickly withdraw the drug.

:: OFF-LABEL MARKETING

When the FDA approves a new treatment, it approves it for a given indication. Atorvastatin is approved to treat various sorts of high cholesterol in various situations. Phenytoin is approved to treat seizures. Once approved, however, these drugs may be prescribed by doctors for other indications. If a doctor wants to prescribe phenytoin for hair loss, she can. This may seem odd but in some cases is reasonable. As we discuss in chapter 18, it is sometimes necessary for doctors to use treatments not supported by a robust evidence base. There are treatments that we have used for years for indications for which they have not been approved. Why have they not been approved? Sometimes there is little incentive to study an intervention because the efficacy seems apparent but there is little prospect for money to be made from it. (No one will pay for a trial if there is no prospect for large returns.) Sometimes drug development and clinical experience proceed faster than the evidence base. Clinicians recognize that a drug is effective before robust trials are designed and completed. Neither of these situations is ideal, but they are the reality. As long as the doctor prescribing a drug for an off-label use is doing so with knowledge of the evidence (or lack thereof) and the patient is well informed, this approach is acceptable. The doctor prescribing phenytoin for hair growth would need to know that there are no data that the drug regrows hair and would need to inform the patient of this fact. Whether insurance companies—and, indirectly, all of us—should pay for these remedies is another question entirely.

What is not acceptable is for a drug company to develop a drug for one indication and then market it for something else. This is the classic bait-and-switch, and it is not rare. In this situation a pharmaceutical company wins approval for a drug for an indication for which it clearly works. Then the company tries to persuade doctors to use it for another indication in order to sell more product. Usually, the indication they promote it for is far more common than the one for which it won approval. In some instances, approval for the new indication may follow a year or two later and no harm is done. In other instances we find that the drug really does not work for the new indication and we have another example of reversal—doctors have been persuaded to use an ineffective drug.

The story of gabapentin is not the most recent, but it is certainly the most egregious example of this practice. In 1993 gabapentin, under the trade name Neurontin, was approved by the FDA to be used, in combination with other drugs, for the treatment of seizures. Parke-Davis, the drug's maker, then began to market it to doctors for an impressive number of maladies. A list of these conditions (included in a later Justice Department press release) included bipolar disorder, pain disorders, Lou Gehrig's disease, attention-deficit disorder, migraine, restless-leg syndrome, and seizures—but as a first-line, single-agent treatment. The marketing of gabapentin as a single agent for seizures was particularly outrageous because the FDA had actually rejected the company's application for this indication.

The aggressive marketing initially paid off—Parke-Davis sold a lot of gabapentin. But in the end, the firm was hit with a $430 million settlement by the Justice Department.* More than 20 years later, gabapentin is still not approved for most of the indications for which it was initially promoted. It is unknown how many patients were harmed because they received a treatment that did not work, experienced adverse effects of gabapentin, or were delayed in their receipt of other, approved treatments for their condition.

::

The roots of reversal are extensive. Primarily, these roots are made of insufficient or flawed data. Often the treatments that are fed by these roots are accepted with the best intentions—doctors and drug and device developers truly believe in the treatments and think the data, or explanatory model, they have are sufficient. This chapter has explored instances when the intentions are less than admirable. Drug developers have willfully distorted evidence in order to sell medications. Guidelines recommend therapies not because they work but because the recommendations serve the interests of the people who wrote the guidelines. Therapies that are approved based on their promise are often not adequately tested. If these therapies are tested and found wanting, they often remain available. It is difficult and expensive to develop a new treatment. It takes dedicated researchers to determine whether a novel therapy is effective. A system riddled with conflicts of interest makes it nearly impossible for the process to work.

---

* This fee was likely much smaller than the profits reaped through off-label promotion—in other words, not large enough to truly serve as a disincentive.

13

WHY ARE WE SO ATTRACTED TO FLAWED THERAPIES?

RECENTLY, A PHYSICIAN FRIEND and insomniac confided in us that the FDA was messing up (not actually her original choice of words). She had read about a new sleep medication, suvorexant, which works not by causing drowsiness but by decreasing wakefulness. Regulators needed to hurry up and approve that medication, she said, because she desperately needed it. Although the comment should not have been surprising, it was. First, being a physician, our friend should know that the "decreasing wakefulness" effect was almost certainly a marketing ploy, being no different from causing drowsiness and not readily assessed by science. Second, she likely also knew that approved sleep aids offer quite minimal benefits.* But even though our physician friend should know all this, she still felt like— hurry up and give me access to that pill. What was wrong with her? It just so happens to be the same thing that is wrong with all of us.

---

* The nonbenzodiazepine hypnotics are the newest and most successful sleep aids presently on the market. Eszopiclone (Lunesta), one of these drugs, earned about $225 million in the fourth quarter of 2013 alone. A recent meta-analysis showed that, on average, these drugs get you to sleep only about 22 minutes faster.

Throughout this book we have given examples of how doctors and patients are seduced by practices that do not work. The phenomenon is ubiquitous—in chapter 7 we argued that as much as 40 percent of the things doctors do are ineffective. In the last few chapters, we have tried to summarize why reversal is so common. Thus far, we have explained the cause of reversal from a scientific standpoint: reversals occur when a practice is adopted before it has a strong evidence base. The weak evidence base is often ignored because of doctors' faith in mechanistic explanations or studies that were designed to be deceptive by industry. The perverse financial incentives among doctors and inventors òften assist the process. But, despite this explanation, we have not tackled the harder problem: what is it that makes us so readily seduced? This is a subtle distinction. To some extent we have dwelled on the how, but there is also a why. Why is it that we, as doctors and patients, are so likely to adopt flawed therapies, even if we understand what makes the promise of a specific novel therapy dubious. Why was our friend so confident that the next new pill would be so great? What is it about us that makes us ready and willing (if not eager) to adopt therapies that may not help?

ACT NOW, DATA LATER

We have a problem; we need a solution. We hear the mantra every day. We need to solve this problem now. Ten minutes ago. Yesterday. It is not just in medicine but everywhere. Global warming, immigration, the federal deficit, obesity. We have to do something now. The problems cited are often serious and real and sometimes truly frightening. Obesity now contributes to one in five deaths in America. Absolutely, it is serious, and absolutely, we need to do whatever we can to reduce the burden of disease. Ridding the country (the world) of obesity cannot come a minute too soon. But what exactly do we do?

Do we promote diet and exercise? Do we concentrate only on the most obese or on those with medical problems resulting from their obesity, or do we try to shift the entire bell curve? Do we change farm subsidies? Do we tax sugar-sweetened beverages? Do we encourage personal responsibility, or corporate responsibility, or both? Do we tell people to eat at home? Does organic help? Does weight depend more on diet or exercise, fat or carbohydrates? When you get to proposing an actual intervention, things get very complicated. Knowing that obesity, HIV, cancer, heart disease, malaria, domestic violence, and suicide are problems is easy. Figuring out how to solve the problems is very hard.

At one of the hospitals where we work, a group recently launched a "stand up once an hour initiative" based on data that time spent sitting is linked to obesity and early death. This "act now" group felt that enough was enough. If you must sit, stand once an hour. Of course, that recommendation has not been tested at all, and posting "stand up" flyers (the actual intervention here) is even further removed from the actual science. It is unlikely that all of the posters and fliers printed—completely well-intentioned—changed any health outcomes. But we live in an "act now" world.

Medical reversal occurs when we act before we have data. Something seems like it should work, so we act on our assumptions. One way of satisfying our need to act, without doing so prematurely, might be to redirect our energy from "act now, data later" to "data now, act later." This could be accomplished by doing exactly what you were going to do anyway: institute your "stand up every hour" initiative, but take 10 percent of the funds you planned to spend on the intervention and use it instead to pay for data collection. Enlist participants and randomize them to stand once an hour or not, and measure weights before and after the study. Better still, randomize medical schools to the placement of posters and fliers and follow the weights of a random sample of students, faculty, and staff before and after. This design is called a "cluster randomized trial." Or be really ambitious and recognize that weight is just a surrogate end point. Can you test whether once-per-hour standing at work will improve quality of life or decrease the incidence of disease or mortality? Yes, it is hard to test an intervention on young people and wait decades for an outcome, so why not pick a high-risk group? Enroll patients in a heart failure clinic and randomize them to stand once an hour. Can you improve clinically important outcomes in this vulnerable population with a simple intervention?

It feels good to do something about a problem, but what is important is to do something that works. "Data now, act later" could actually prove efficacy, thus providing a real solution to the problem.

THE TECHNOLOGY EFFECT

Another reason we are so attracted to flawed therapies is the obviousness of the benefits of technology. Over the past century, technology has successfully addressed problems that, historically, seemed intractable. We now communicate and travel around the world with ease. We are freed from the discomfort of hot summer days and cold winter nights. Information is now available anytime, anywhere. Just 25 years ago, disputes about basic facts—for instance, was Kevin Bacon in *Apollo 13*?—could not be answered until the library (or the video store) opened the next day. Now, there is no reason to speculate.

Because technology has addressed so many of our daily challenges, we are eager to embrace the next innovation. But, as we discussed in chapter 10, not every advance that would seem to offer obvious benefit really does. Sometimes we do not need a study to tell us whether a new technology is better than the old one; sometimes we do; and this helps explain why we are so vulnerable to reversal. When it comes to your new iPhone or television, you do not need a randomized trial to tell you that the screen is crisper, the processor is smoother, and the sound is clearer. Because of this, we come to believe that the new sleeping pill must be better than the old one, or that a prostatectomy performed by a robot must be better than one performed by a surgeon. But the human body is very different from technology. It is much more complicated and more challenging (as well as more magnificent). Its complete workings remain largely a mystery, and the effects of our interventions are often small, below the sensitivity of crude human observation. You cannot observe two surgical approaches and know which is better the way you can view two TVs and choose the superior one. And yet, the temptation to extrapolate our experiences with technology to biology is irresistible.

Whatever the reason, our tendency to believe that "newer is better" is real. Focus groups of health-care consumers reveal this bias.* In one study, not only did people believe that newer technology was usually better, but one-third also felt that medical treatments that work the best usually cost the most. Only one-third of participants recalled having a physician explain the scientific evidence that shows which care is best. Many surveyed were unclear what "evidence" even is—thinking it was the totality of their test results and exam findings and not the studies that support the benefit of an intervention.

---

* Increasingly, patients are being called consumers or clients, and doctors are called providers. These are terms we have assiduously avoided.

DIRECT-TO-CONSUMER ADVERTISING

In America, it is not just our predispositions that lead us to believe in new technologies; we also have a little help in the form of direct-to-consumer (DTC) advertising, advertisements produced by drug companies and shown to potential patients. No matter how little media you consume, you are certainly familiar with the nearly ubiquitous advertisements for the newest drugs. They appear on TV, radio, and Internet pop-ups. The United States is one of only two nations that permit the DTC marketing of medical products. Besides being annoyed by some of the advertisements, many people do not see a problem with DTC advertising of prescription drugs. Admittedly, the advertisements create interest in a new, generally more expensive product, but proponents assert that the advertisements are also educational, and if a person still needs to ask his doctor for a prescription, what is the problem?

In 2005 a group of researchers nicely illustrated why we should worry about DTC advertising. They performed a randomized trial in which they enlisted standardized patients (SPs). SPs are actors who are trained to convincingly play the part of a patient. In this study, SPs were sent to visit local general practitioners and were randomized to display one of two disorders: depression or adjustment disorder. We all know what depression is, a serious mental illness that is often, appropriately, treated with medications. Adjustment disorder is on the depression spectrum; it resembles depression but is generally milder. It occurs when the normal reaction to a real life trauma—the loss of a job or a loved one—becomes excessive. Adjustment disorder occurs when life stressors overwhelm our coping ability. The treatment is generally time and counseling, not medications.

In the trial, each SP was randomized to describe depression or adjustment disorder. The SPs were also randomized to make one of three types of requests of the physicians: brand-specific; general; or none. The brand-specific request was something like "I recently saw an ad for Paxil, might it help me?" The generic request was "Could I benefit from a medication?" The results were intriguing on multiple levels. First, advertisers got what they paid for: if an SP made a brand-specific request, she was much more likely to receive the brand of medication she requested. Second, if an SP requested a medication, she was more likely to get one than if she did not. Third, the SPs who made any type of request were more likely to receive appropriate care than those who did not. Thus, being an informed patient helps us to get the best care, and being an informed patient who has been told by a drug company what to ask for helps the drug company. Among s Ps presenting with symptoms of adjustment disorder, a condition usually not treated with medication, 10 percent who did not make a request left with a prescription—probably an appropriate proportion. For those who made a general or brand-specific request, the prescribing rates were 39 and 55 percent, respectively.

These results tell us just why drug companies love D T C advertising. The ads do two things. First, they "educate" the public that medications exist, and, second, they provide specific brand names. Even though a doctor is the ultimate gatekeeper, when patients bring up drugs and specific brands to doctors, they often get what they ask for. After all, there is a lot of art to medicine, and as a general rule, unless the request is completely off the mark, it pays to work with patients.

Between 1999 and 2005, D T C advertising increased from just under $1 billion to just over $4 billion. This increase tells you that D T C marketing successfully sells drugs. Does it also work to improve health? Unfortunately, we do not know. While it might seem draconian to restrict the ability of companies to advertise their products, prescription drugs are a different commodity from Caribbean vacations or new cars. You need a great deal of training to make sense of the studies that evaluate new drugs and to impartially conclude when they are best used. Laws that require motorcycle helmets, seatbelts, and contributions to the social security program exist because people do not always weigh risk appropriately. As a society, we believe that, to an extent, a role of government is to protect people from unnecessarily risky or bad decisions. D T C advertising is good for business but may not be good for health. For these reasons, D T C advertising remains banned in every country except the United States and New Zealand.

BASIC SCIENCE IN EDUCATION

"Act now, data later," the technology effect, and advertising influence the choices of people outside the medical field as much as they do people inside it. The next couple of topics preferentially influence doctors and how they make patient-care decisions. One reason doctors are so easily swayed by the newest breakthrough in the medical sciences is that mechanistic thinking is so deeply engrained in our training. In medical school, the study of how therapies should work is much more extensive and comes before the study of whether therapies do work. In other words, we would much rather quiz medical students about whether venlafaxine inhibits postsynaptic reuptake of norepinephrine, serotonin, or both, than ask them to critically appraise the randomized trials testing whether, and to what extent, venlafaxine improves depressive symptoms. If that sounds odd—it is. Our current system is a result of how medical knowledge and education have evolved. For most of the 20th century, quizzing medical students about how things should work was all medical schools could do. There was a paucity of trials testing whether and to what extent therapies actually did work. Then the evidence-based movement began, and clinical practice shifted, but education has been slow to follow.

When we talk about how therapies should work, we are talking about the basic sciences. We are talking about the mechanisms of how things work. In the scientific tradition, there are two complementary schools of thought, reductionism and empiricism. Reductionists believe that the more we understand about the mechanism by which disease happens and therapies act, the closer we are to optimally targeting therapy and curing disease. Empiricists are concerned foremost with whether interventions work. Why should you give a drug in the angiotensin-converting enzyme-inhibitor class to a patient with heart failure? The reductionist would answer, Because it prevents ventricular remodeling (a maladaptive process). The empiricist would answer, because multiple randomized trials show that it improves outcomes. You see the distinction? The views are complementary. You have to be a reductionist to have a good understanding of biology and to drive medical innovation. But in the end, it is the empiricist whose answer is correct. However, historically, the reductionist approach has always had priority in medical education.

Doctors who care for patients should be, and mostly are, empiricists. We are happy to use drugs that have been shown to work even though we do not quite understand their mechanisms of action. For instance, we know inhaled anesthetic gases can knock you out, but we have no idea just how they work. The training in premedical courses and in medical school, however, is heavily steeped in reductionism. We learn organic chemistry and biochemistry. We learn molecular biology. We learn anatomy. All of this understanding is important—to a certain extent. If you are planning to have a career developing new drugs, then it is very important. But the internist who writes a prescription for a blood-pressure pill does not really care a whole lot about how it works; he cares that it lowers blood pressure (a surrogate end point) and decreases cardiovascular events (a clinically important end point). Even a surgeon is most concerned with the few dozen anatomic structures she crosses paths with—she has long forgotten the thousands of tiny tendrils she dissected in anatomy class. It is for this reason that empiricism should carry the day in medical training.

Rather than being replaced, reductionism is experiencing a revival. When people celebrate the coming era of "personalized medicine," they imply that soon our understanding of the mechanism of disease will be so robust, so sophisticated, that you will not need to empirically demonstrate the efficacy of interventions. This is unrealistically optimistic. Whether the mechanism for a therapy is the mechanics of lung inflation or the tiny binding pocket of a renegade protein, you still need a trial to ensure that what you are doing actually accomplishes the ends you envision. The rumors of empiricism's demise have been greatly exaggerated.

For an editorial in the *Journal of the American Medical Association,* Arthur Slutsky, a well-respected critical-care physician, used the subtitle "The Seduction of Physiology." What did he mean? Slutsky understood that doctors like interventions that cause improvements in vital measures like blood pressure and oxygenation. We know these numbers are important, are objective, and correspond to improvements in physiology that we understand. It is reasonable to assume that if we can improve these measures in critically ill patients, we can improve survival. Therein lies the false seduction of physiology. Many times, we have found that interventions that improve these measures do nothing to improve the survival of the patient. Improving physiological measures is comforting, but it does not always affect outcomes. None of this is to say that paying attention to physiology or designing therapies that improve physiological measures is worthless—it is not. But any such intervention must be rigorously tested, rather than blindly followed. In the next chapter we propose a system of medical education that does a better job of balancing the importance of empiricism and reductionism.

ABANDONING A PAYCHECK

A colleague recently joked that flawed therapies have paid for many a beach house. His statement is cynical and hyperbolic but not without truth. In chapter 8, we wrote about how tenaciously interventional cardiologists have clung to the practice of stenting open coronary lesions in people with stable angina—a $12 billion a year industry—even after the COURAGE trial showed it was ineffective. Sure, interventional cardiologists have witnessed cases in which these stents have benefited patients, but they are also the group most likely to have their income negatively impacted by the findings of COURAGE.

Although doctors—ourselves included—like to believe that no amount of financial remuneration could sway their judgment, hundreds of studies have shown that financial conflicts of interest do bias physicians. When you hear of conflict of interest, you might think of doctors doing consulting work. A psychiatrist is paid by Merck to give talks on depression and then goes on to emphasize the benefits of Merck drugs. This certainly is a conflict, but it is one that our field has been pretty aggressive in exposing. We wish we had a nickel for every "COI form" we have completed before giving talks or publishing papers. However, there are far more insidious types of conflict of interest. Any time a physician recommends a procedure or treatment that will increase his take-home pay, there is at least the potential for conflict of interest. Orthopedists may not always see the downside of joint replacement as clearly as nonorthopedists; oncologists tend to err on the side of giving chemotherapy; and general internists who own X-ray machines tend to order more X-rays. A recent study tracked urology specialists' groups that bought a machine that could deliver radiation to the prostate. Are you surprised that groups that purchased the machine tended to give more radiation?

It is very hard to accept evidence that something you have done for patients, something that you truly believed was beneficial, is not useful. The evidence is even harder to accept when you have been well compensated for your work. Because of this, acceptance of medical reversals is never easy and opposition to them is usually passionate.

::

Human beings are creative, optimistic, and hopeful. These are traits that have served our species well. At the same time, these traits make us susceptible to medical reversals. Our creative minds figure out ways that therapies may work—what intracellular pathways they would affect, what principles of physiology they satisfy. Our optimistic side feels better, even when interventions are equivalent to the placebo. In our hopefulness we continue to believe that tomorrow will be better than today. The enduring belief is that the new and more expensive must be better than the old and economical. In many aspects of life, this disposition is surely beneficial—we make more friends, solve problems, and enjoy ourselves—but when it comes to deciding how to plan our health-care systems and how to manage our own medical care, these traits can lead to erroneous conclusions. In the next chapters we argue that although the roots of reversal are vast, from the scientific method to human psychology, a few simple rules can curb its growth and even prune it back.

PART 4

BEYOND REVERSAL

14
MEDICAL EDUCATION
:: A VERY GOOD PLACE TO START

OVER THE COURSE of this book, we have sought to answer the questions, how often are accepted practices overturned (reversed, not replaced)? and, why does reversal occur? We have presented the case that reversal is ubiquitous in medical practice and its causes are diverse. These include financial bias, investigator bias, and unbridled (and unjustified) optimism with regard to novel treatments on the part of all the players in medicine: doctors, scientists, industry, fledgling biotech companies, advocacy groups, the media, and patients. Our next step is to move from theory to practice. If we accept that reversal is common, harmful, and not a necessary part of medical progress, can we find a way to decrease its prevalence?

With such diverse causes, it will be a challenge to end, or even reduce, reversal. We need to find a bottleneck, a narrow canyon, where all the sources can be ambushed. Thankfully, we have such a place. Because the proximate cause of reversal is adopting therapies based on insufficient evidence, improving evidence will reduce the prevalence of medical reversal.

How do we improve the evidence on which the practice of medicine is based? In theory, it seems pretty simple. For all new medical practices, screening tests, diagnostic tests, pills, novel devices, procedures, and surgeries, well-done randomized trials must show improvement in real outcomes (such as quality of life or mortality) before those practices gain FDA approval or are widely used. Instituting this strategy would ensure that all new practices really work and might even check the rising costs of medicine by no longer spending money on ineffective innovations. We also need to address the existing therapies that lack a strong evidence base. To do this, we could enumerate all existing, unproved medical practices and rank them by cost and frequency of use. Then, prioritizing the common and costly ones, test each with a randomized trial. We would then abandon whatever does not work. John McKinlay, whom we spoke of earlier, was truly prescient when he suggested similar solutions 35 years ago.

If only it were really that simple. To implement such a solution, the entire health-care industry would require a new ethic. This ethic would demand that the burden of proof, the task of proving the utility of every new therapy (and the older, unproven ones), rest on those who stand to benefit from instituting the therapy. The implementation of this strategy would be challenged by a long list of reasonable concerns. How would we stimulate (or legislate) the adoption of a new ethic? Would requiring more solid evidence before adopting new therapies slow innovation? What would count as solid evidence? Certainly not every randomized controlled trial is a good one. What sorts of end points should randomized trials examine? And why should we not just throw out all unproven medicine in one fell swoop?

We try to answer these concerns in the coming chapters. But first, in this chapter and the next, we suggest some specific reforms that we think would go a long way toward changing the culture of medicine. We start where doctors start, in medical school, and then move to where many doctors are trained and where much of the medical innovation occurs, in academic medical sciences.

These chapters are quite different from the preceding ones. Up to this point we have taken great care to support everything we have said with evidence. When we pointed out a reversal, we outlined how the therapy was proved to be ineffective and explained why, in retrospect, doctors had mistakenly accepted the therapy. These chapters are, by necessity, more speculative. We cannot say for sure that a certain type of medical training, or a certain standard for promotion of academic faculty, increases the prevalence of reversal. Furthermore, we certainly cannot know that the reforms we suggest would reduce the frequency of reversal in the future. But we

explain why we believe certain features of medical education and the structure of academic medical centers predispose our field to accepting therapies that are later overturned. We then go on to suggest changes that we
think will be effective but that we hope will be tested. We would obviously
be the last people to suggest that an intervention be accepted just because
it makes sense.

WHAT MAKES A GOOD PHYSICIAN?

When we consider how doctors should be trained, we need to think first
about the sort of doctor we want to produce. We need to get very specific
here—we need to specify who the *we* is when we ask, What type of doctors do *we* want? Medical schools are interested in graduating fine physicians and academic leaders (which often means doctors who are most productive in research). All other things being equal, they prefer to turn out
doctors who generously support the alumni association. Residency direc-
tors have a shorter horizon when considering the medical school product.
A resident who works hard, furthers the hospital's clinical mission, gains
admission to a prestigious fellowship, and does not cause problems is the
ideal doctor for a training program. Hospital systems and medical groups
are looking for "rainmakers," those doctors who can bring in many grants
or well-insured patients, ideally for highly reimbursed treatments. Payers,
on the other hand, are hoping for doctors who are cost-conscious, ordering few tests and making fewer referrals. We could, of course, go on to talk
about the desires of plaintiffs' lawyers, defense lawyers, and pharmaceutical companies.

For our purposes, let us consider the sort of doctors that we, as future
patients, want. Of course there is no one type of doctor that every person
wants. The doctors we desire are as diverse as we are. Some of us want a
doctor who will give us full autonomy in our decision making, while others want a doctor who will strongly guide us. We have worked with doctors
who are warm and friendly and others who seem distant and detached. We
have known doctors who refer to their patients by first names and always
ask about patients' families, travels, and holidays and others who expressly
steer clear of these perceived niceties. All these doctors have had loyal cad-
res of patients.

What then can we say about the doctors we want our medical schools to
produce? Tomorrow's doctor probably needs to master three areas while

in medical school: the doctor-patient relationship, systems-based practice, and practice-based learning. First, the doctor-patient relationship. While no doctor can be everything to everybody, it is not asking too much that our schools train their graduates to be most things to most patients. They must interpret a patient's needs and values and respond in a productive, therapeutic manner. They need to understand how to communicate with all types of people: those who want autonomy and those who do not; those who want a hand-holder and those who want a more distant, though empathic, guide; those who look like the doctor and those who do not. To develop this kind of physician requires schools to provide extensive mentored clinical experience.

Not only do our doctors need to be experts in working with patients; they need to work within the growing health-care team in a facile manner. Decades ago doctors collaborated only with nurses (and often in less-than-collegial ways). Today, every hospitalization requires that the attending physician work collaboratively not only with nurses but with subspecialty teams, physical therapists, social workers, case managers, and many other affiliated health-care workers. In today's lingo, this is referred to as systems-based practice.

Lastly, we want doctors to know their stuff. They cannot be satisfied with "knowing their stuff" when they graduate, since most of the specific "stuff" they learned will be obsolete before they complete their training. Tomorrow's doctors need to master the skills necessary to practice from a strong and current evidence base throughout their careers. This means continuing to learn from their patients and from the medical literature until the day they retire. We call this practice-based learning. Doctors need to interpret data so that they know which interventions are well supported and which are not, and then be able to present this information to their patients. Medical school graduates who enter careers in research must be motivated to always question untested dogma. Physician scientists need to think not only like scientists but like clinicians as well.

RETHINKING THE FOUNDATIONS
OF MEDICAL EDUCATION

Although we train many extraordinary doctors, the frequency of reversal in medicine tells us that, at present, our system of medical education is not completely successful. Medical education stands on two pillars, constructed in the early 20th century. The first pillar is premedical (college) course work. Many of these courses, such as organic chemistry, physics, and calculus, are the subjects that were important in the early 1900s. (These courses were probably deemed important at that time because they were the only subjects with any bearing on the study of medicine.) The second pillar is the four-year medical-school curriculum: years one and two spent studying science and years three and four spent seeing patients. This was the groundbreaking approach to structuring medical education put forth by Abraham Flexner in the early 1900s.

Today, both of these pillars of training are being questioned. Critics argue that the college classes students take to gain acceptance to medical school are of little (organic chemistry) or no (physics and calculus) use to the practicing physician. These courses not only do little to prepare students for their careers as doctors; they are not even necessary to understand the first two years (the science portion) of medical school. Furthermore, the first two years of studying science in medical school have been criticized as being of little value to the vast majority of physicians.

If we accept these critiques, premedical and medical education should be reformed for the sake of efficiency alone. However, we have an even deeper concern about the structure of medical education. It is not hard to see that the years spent studying how the body's small parts work may actually be harmful. These classes indoctrinate students with a belief in the primacy of the foundational medical sciences over the clinical ones. As we noted in chapter 13, we currently train students to be reductionists rather than empiricists. Students come to believe that a medical therapy works because of its mechanism. This is not an absolute truth. The mechanism is one way a therapy might work. If the same model explains future data, then it is probably the way this therapy does work. One can only be certain that a given therapy actually works when the therapy is shown to work in randomized controlled trials.

Science is the theory that underlies medicine. Science (as well as experience) is crucial for generating hypotheses to be tested. Clinical trials are real-world data points. Let us consider the example of cholesterol-lowering medications in the treatment of high cholesterol. The hypothesis suggested that because high cholesterol is associated with heart attacks, lowering cholesterol would prevent heart attacks. Trials using statin-type cholesterol-lowering drugs were designed to test this hypothesis. The trials proved that using statins prevents heart attacks. The trials did not prove the success of the mechanism (in this case, that lowering cholesterol prevents heart attacks). It will take more trials, with other types of medications, to prove the mechanism. This has not yet been done. In many other cases, the hypothesis is actually disproved, leaving us with neither a mechanism nor a viable treatment. Recall the CAST trial from chapter 1. In that example the mechanism that was proposed was that decreasing the frequency of premature ventricular contractions would save lives. When this was tested, we found that the hypothesis was incorrect and the treatment based on it was actually harmful. Proponents of scientific models are sometimes so confident that they regard trials as a nuisance.

Thus, the problem in the organization of medical education is a problem of priority. It is not that basic science is unnecessary to physicians and that medical students should never learn or think about it. Absolutely not. Without a rich understanding of the foundational sciences, medical progress would cease. But basic science is not the first thing a practicing clinician should learn. The primacy of the basic sciences is the reason that cardiologists could not accept the finding that niacin did not save lives. It is why radiologists could not accept that vertebroplasty did not help back pain. It is the reason orthopedists could not accept that repairing torn menisci did not help knee pain. They thought, "How can an empirical study contradict the mechanism?" The reality is that the human body is so complicated, and our understanding of it so superficial, that what we believe should work often does not.

REBUILDING MEDICAL EDUCATION
FROM THE GROUND UP

What, then, should a medical education that is designed to produce better clinicians, less prone to advocating ineffective treatments, look like? This training would start before medical school. A student committed to becoming a doctor should be expected to arrive at medical school already knowing the basics of biochemistry and physiology (the chemical and molecular basis of all life). An understanding of basic anatomy would also be expected. Anatomic studies have traditionally been reserved for the rarified (and formaldehyde-infused) air of medical schools, based on the idea that the privilege of dissecting the human cadaver should be reserved for physicians in training. In today's world of lifelike models and three-dimensional computer imaging, there is no reason that college students could not take part in high-quality anatomy courses. A strong argument could be made that understanding how our bodies work, on both a microscopic and a macroscopic level, is not out of place in a 21st-century college education. This preliminary course work (biochemistry, physiology, anatomy) is certainly teachable in undergraduate and postbaccalaureate programs. It should take the place of the currently required courses (physics, calculus) that were considered critical preparation for medical school around the time of the First World War.

Once students arrive in medical school, there would still be preclinical studies, but these would be radically altered to what we call an "encounter-based model," in which the entire curriculum would build from the patient encounter. (A "map" of our proposed curriculum is shown in figure 14.1 at the end of the chapter.) Every patient-doctor interaction begins with the patient's concerns: What is my diagnosis? How will you treat me? What can I/we do so that I remain well? For each concern, students would learn to differentiate the relevant history from information that is merely distraction. They would learn which physical findings are most diagnostic, which diagnostic tests are most effective to accurately rank the list of possible diagnoses, and which treatments are most effective, based on real, clinical evidence. These early clinical encounters would begin to train students to become the doctors we need and want. Not only would they learn to practice truly evidence-based medicine; they would also learn how to work with all patients and function as part of the team that delivers today's medical care.

In an encounter-based model, the traditional preclinical courses would be abandoned as students learned how to manage patient encounters from a foundation of empiricism rather than from scientific theory that may or may not explain how or why interventions work. The curriculum would include instruction in clinical reasoning and decision making, techniques to search the medical literature, and critical appraisal of medical studies. Other courses would familiarize students with landmark clinical trials and biostatistical concepts as well as giving instruction in how to make clinical decisions when the existing evidence base is weak. An encounter-based curriculum would immediately put to use textbooks that are presently not used until the clinical years. This would be appropriate because students would be learning the skills of differential diagnosis, evaluation, and treatment—skills essential for a practicing physician—from nearly day one of medical school. Students would begin with the most common complaints diagnosed and managed by generalists and gradually move to the less common diagnoses—those usually managed by specialists. The tempo of these courses would be slow at first, allowing educators both to assure that students' scientific knowledge base is adequate and to provide a foundation in the language of the science of medicine. Similar to today's curricula, the preclinical period would culminate with an intensive study of pathophysiology. However, in this revised curriculum, the study of pathophysiology would teach students scientific models not as a justification for how medicine is practiced but as a basis to understand the current theory of disease.

This preliminary course work could be completed in 12 months, allowing for expanded and revised clinical education. The goals of the clinical years are threefold, reflecting our three goals for our graduates. Students would learn to develop effective patient-doctor relationships, to work within a complicated and ever-evolving clinical team, and to master clinical reasoning—the ability to work from a patient's symptom to an accurate diagnosis, using the tools of the medical history, the physical exam, and appropriately acquired and interpreted diagnostic tests. During the clinical years, students would also master the most evidence-based therapeutics, both medical and surgical.

Presently, the clinical years of medical school are essentially an apprenticeship. Students rotate with senior physicians and are trained by these doctors. The learning in the various specialties (obstetrics and gynecology, surgery, pediatrics, and so forth) is enhanced by didactic curricula meant to fill the holes in the clinical experience. This method has historically been effective—American medical schools produce fine physicians—but inefficient; not all mentors are equally skilled, and students often master topics that are uncommon, thus providing little benefit to their future patients, at the expense of more common, fundamental problems.

The expanded clinical years in a reformed system would carry both greater demands and greater potential. In this proposed curriculum, some of the medical sciences that are currently covered in the "preclinical biennium" would be taught. These topics could now be focused and relevant, being closely linked to clinical cases. In our quest to decrease medical reversal, time would be spent in small groups learning to critically evaluate the evidence behind every decision made during an actual patient encounter.

Students would learn to care for today's patient while mastering the skills needed for lifelong learning. This structure would actually benefit patient care in the training environment. Imagine mentored students in hospitals and medical clinics who work at vetting the diagnostic approach and therapy being offered to patients for the adequacy of its evidence base. With the core clinical experience expanded from 12 to 18 months, there would be ample time to achieve these goals.

In the current model of medical education, the 12 months following the core clinical rotations is the fourth year of medical school, characterized recently by one of our medical students as a very expensive vacation. In our proposed, reformed system, the 18 months that follow the core clinical rotations could be used to enhance the skills and knowledge that students had been acquiring. What would the student have learned? At this point in her training, this "senior student" would possess a relevant and practical knowledge of the scientific foundation of medicine, clinical skills, and an intuitive understanding of the evidence on which practice is based, as well as a pretty good idea of what she wants do to for the rest of her career.

What would we do in these final 18 months? First, to put the encounter-based curriculum in place, we reduced preclinical science training. Now, after the student has been grounded in clinical and evidence-based medicine, is the perfect time to teach the basic sciences. Physiology, cell biology, pharmacology, and other foundational sciences could be revisited at this time. Teaching these sciences to students who already know clinical medicine would be revolutionary. Students at this point would be junior clinicians, rather than recent college graduates, so the instruction could be clinically relevant and case-based. Furthermore, because these students would understand the applicability of the subject matter to clinical medicine, their motivation to learn the material would be enhanced. Because the detailed basic science education would follow experience with trial-based decision making, students would be unlikely to trust mechanistic explanations as the basis for therapy—one common cause of reversals.

Beyond the basic science courses, students could pursue courses and clinical experiences most applicable to their chosen disciplines in medicine. Besides the currently offered clinical rotations, in which students take on more clinical responsibilities and work with subspecialist consultants, there would be a range of seminar, laboratory, clinical simulation, and didactic courses: intensive anatomy for surgeons; advanced diagnostic reasoning for future internists; advanced training in translational research for those hoping to become medical scientists.

OVERCOMING THE CRITICS

As with any curriculum revision, the naysayers will be numerous. Their objections are easy to predict. First, they will say that such restructuring would be hard to adopt. In reality, the only difficult challenge would be having medical schools agree on prerequisites. These discussions are already under way. In addition, if the most competitive medical schools, those that admit a tiny fraction of applicants, begin to publicize their new admission requirements, students will work to satisfy them. It will take some brave medical school and university deans to be the first to adopt such a strategy, but medical schools function in a seller's market. Many of the nation's newest medical schools (the Cleveland Clinic Lerner College of Medicine and the University of Central Florida College of Medicine) have adopted progressive curricula with no shortage of applicants.

Others might argue that the requirement of more advanced science classes in the undergraduate years would make it more difficult for non–science majors, who are increasingly attractive to medical schools, to enter medicine. In reality the number of requirements might decrease as the type of courses changes. If more students do end up needing to complete their undergraduate course work after college, medical schools (and patients) will only benefit from applicants who are a little older, a little more mature, and a little more committed to their medical education.

The loudest objection might be that if basic scientific training is decreased, there will be little that differentiates physicians from physician assistants and nurse practitioners. The argument might be that sacrificing training in the scientific foundation of medicine will leave physicians practicing from algorithms. Critics might say that tomorrow's doctors would be unable to reason from the pathophysiology that underlies the most complicated cases. In fact, we believe the new structure would actually enhance physicians' scientific knowledge. The more tightly scientific learning and clinical learning are integrated, the more applicable this knowledge will be to the care of patients. In the reformed system, students would learn the foundational sciences from a team of clinicians and basic scientists teaching the most clinically relevant sciences. This differs from the present standard, in which the basic sciences are typically taught by scientists, often gifted in their fields but just as often having little connection to the world of the clinic. These teachers are often likely to teach what they study and enjoy rather than what is critical to the physician in training.

Maybe most convincing in our argument for reform is that some of our finest and most progressive medical schools are already moving in this direction. Many schools no longer require applicants to take college math but suggest biochemistry. Duke University School of Medicine, one of the first to break with Flexnerian dogma, reduced preclinical training to one year. This unified year includes integrated courses in the science of health and disease (rather than the standard curriculum in which students learn about the healthy body in year one and the diseased body in year two). Although Duke made these changes to allow more time for research training, the new program has shown that reduced preclinical training is compatible with training excellent physicians. Many other fine schools, including Yale, Harvard, Case Western Reserve, and Columbia, have either recently reduced, or are planning to reduce, the length of their preclinical curriculum. This curricular change is becoming so common that it seems less and less remarkable. The schools each have their own reasons for making the change, but their willingness to alter their curricula argues that major changes can be made.

Some schools have gone even further. New York University School of Medicine is the first school to offer a medical degree in three years. Selected students are able to complete the preclinical course work in 18 months with a curriculum more focused on their chosen specialty. Texas Tech Health Science Center School of Medicine, Mercer University School of Medicine, and others are also experimenting with three-year programs.

::

The practice of medicine today would be unrecognizable to the medical student and medical educator of the early 20th century, yet the structure of medical school today is unchanged from this bygone era. Diseases that were common 100 years ago have become rare, while new diseases have emerged. Antibiotics were a dream, the stethoscope was advanced technology, and DNA was decades from discovery. The concept that decision making could be based on large clinical trials did not exist, nor did the idea that the universe of medical information could be accessible at the bedside. Although we train excellent physicians, we do so inefficiently, and our

First Year

Human anatomy	The patient encounter					Pathophysiology
	Finding & understanding medical trials	Medical statistics	Clinical reasoning	Medical decision making	Medical ethics	
	The human body in health (Traditional basic sciences)					

Core Clinical: 18 months

	Mentored clinical decision making								
Elective time	Psychiatry	Emergency medicine	Family medicine	Medicine	Surgery	Pediatrics	Obstetrics & gynecology	Neurology	Radiology

Post Clinical Sciences and Specialization: 18 Months

The basic sciences in medicine	Acting internships	Biomedical, clinical, and translational research	Specialty-specific elective time

14.1 Proposed medical school curriculum.

training predisposes these doctors to promote and use therapies that will eventually be found wanting. A reformed system, organized around patient encounters and the analysis of investigative trial data, would train the next generation of physicians to practice a more reliable brand of medicine.

15 ACADEMIC MEDICINE

THUS FAR, WE HAVE DESCRIBED how medical reversal happens and how its harms affect us. We have been writing about what goes on in regular doctors' offices—actually not just offices, but in community hospitals, clinics, and operating rooms across the country. This is where most medicine happens. It is where the doctors who are the workhorses of American medicine care for patients. These doctors dictate how medicine is practiced. Their work is incredibly important and reflects so much of what makes the practice of medicine beautiful. Most aspiring physicians hope to break out on their own and practice their craft in the communities they love.

However, most of what is new in medicine does not come from these physicians. Doctors in the community are too busy to dream up new technologies and drugs, test them, and disseminate their results. By and large, the new things in medicine come from someplace else. They come from the academic medical centers, the so-called Ivory Towers. These centers—places like Johns Hopkins, the Mayo Clinic, the University of Chicago, the Harvard hospitals—are institutions committed not just to patient care but also to advancing research and discovery and training future physicians. They are usually closely affiliated with medical schools and universities. In chapter 14, we proposed that medical schools are a good place to address reversal, since all doctors pass through their halls. In this chapter we turn our attention to the academic medical centers, to see how the incentive structures at these institutions might contribute to reversal—and how altering this structure might reduce the prevalence of reversal.

We will do a lot of speculating here, even more than in the previous chapter. There is little research into how the organization of academic centers affects the staying power of the innovations they produce. What follows comes from our observations and those of our colleagues. Academic medical centers are immensely productive places with amazingly smart people turning out mind-bogglingly innovative research. There are, however, things about these centers that may undermine their excellence, or at least keep them from fully realizing their potential.

SUPERSPECIALISTS

Community physicians, including those who have specialized (becoming cardiologists, allergists, hematologists, hand surgeons) care for a wide breadth of patients. A cardiologist might take care of patients with coronary-artery disease, heart failure, and arrhythmias. An endocrinologist will care for people with osteoporosis, diabetes, thyroid disease, and pituitary tumors. Academic physicians often concentrate on a much narrower range of problems. With the exception of the general physicians who fill out the ranks at these centers (family physicians, pediatricians, and internists), much of the faculty at academic medical centers is made up of superspecialists. They are particularly skilled in very small pieces of the health-care puzzle. You might find a cardiologist who focuses solely on cardiac valves—not the coronary arteries, not the muscle of the heart, not the electrical conduction—just those wonderful, paper-thin flaps of durable tissue that open and close each time your heart beats.

This degree of specialization has been both inevitable and advantageous. Because we know so much more than we did a century ago, and the growth in our knowledge has been so rapid, no single person could ever master all the information even within a single specialty; for the most part, only someone deeply specialized will possess the foundational knowledge necessary to truly innovate. Medical advances depend on superspecialists.

There is, however, a price for this degree of specialization. Doctors who focus on just one problem risk losing perspective, coming to see patients—

and even the whole of medicine—through the narrow lens of their specialty. By definition, these specialists know everything about their field—not
just all the randomized trials ever conducted, but most of the observational
studies and the basic science insights as well. Because of their narrow focus,
and their knowledge of every study (including those of suspect methodol-
ogy), these doctors can become overly committed to a therapy. They insist
that some drug or intervention should be given to a patient, citing the rare
report of improved surrogate end points (not exactly robust evidence). It is
often a challenge for these superspecialists to collaborate clinically. It calls
for quite a degree of thoughtfulness and humility to entertain the valid
input of their (not quite) peers, who may sometimes point out that there
is no good evidence supporting the treatment they endorse. The solution
to the problem created by superspecialists is to include doctors trained in
the big picture, and in assessing evidence-based medicine, when it comes
to making decisions for patients.

THOUGHT LEADERS

A subset of superspecialists become thought leaders in their fields. These
leaders are the people we all—specialists, generalists, the media—rely on
to make the biggest discoveries and to explain how the newest innovations
affect patient care. When a new study about cholesterol therapy is published, one of a dozen or so thought leaders write the editorials in top journals, give nearly all of the interviews in the media, and guide most of the
discussion. If a new study comes out on cancer of the kidney, everyone
wants one New York City doctor's opinion. When it comes to the care of
the elderly, a certain Harvard faculty member is sure to be widely quoted.

How might thought leaders have an impact on medical reversal? At
times, thought leaders charge money to meet with and advise pharmaceutical companies. Sometimes these funds are called honoraria and are presented as a gift for giving a talk or sitting through a meeting. The size of
honoraria can be significant. An important thought leader can make tens of
thousands of dollars (or more) by consulting with drugmakers, insurance
companies, and device manufacturers. The relationship between thought
leaders and the companies that develop treatments is complicated. Not
only does the thought leader provide his advice and opinion to industry.
Industry also gets to describe its vision and argue the merits of its intervention. The relationship is a two-way street.

Receiving money and working so closely with industry is a recipe for corruption. Of course, most thought leaders are not only honest but wholly committed to the best science. The problem is that the influence of industry is subtle. A doctor who spends significant amounts of time with a pharmaceutical company may tend to give the company the benefit of the doubt with its new drug or study. The thought leader may come to believe that the industry is right—maybe that a one-month improvement in survival for a terminal disease is a big deal. A thought leader may hear so many times that "depression is a chemical imbalance" that he begins to favor pharmacotherapy over counseling for all mood disorders. It is hard to believe that thought leaders are not influenced or at all swayed by this work.

The only way to reduce this influence is to keep experts from engaging in these relationships. There have been steps in the right direction. Some universities have set limits on the amount of outside funds that their faculty can receive in this manner. The Physician Payments Sunshine Act took effect in 2013. This act requires manufacturers of drugs and medical devices to track and report certain payments and items of value given to physicians and teaching hospitals. Researchers in the U.S. federal government, such as those at the National Institutes of Health, are forbidden to engage in these practices. This seemingly draconian rule should probably become the norm.

WORKING WITH INDUSTRY

Even if industry does not pay thought leaders for their time, many academic physicians still have to work with for-profit companies. New drugs are often tested across several universities, with money being transferred from companies to the hospitals to help defray the sizable costs of running a trial. To some degree this is inevitable—how can industry conduct trials without academic partnerships? Drug companies do not have direct access to patients. At the same time, such relationships can lead to perverse incentives. Universities become dependent on the substantial income they receive from running trials and thus try to increase the number of trials they conduct. These deeper ties to industry come at a cost as well as a profit. It may be challenging to question the design of trials conducted by a particular pharmaceutical company if your institution's financial health relies on a relationship with that company.

A first step to correct this problem would be to introduce greater transparency into the process. How much money do medical centers make from conducting industry trials? We should also ask whether there should be limits to the proportion of a department's income that can come from industry. Should an oncology department have 30 percent of its revenue come from running trials? 50 percent? How much is too much?

Limits such as these could have a positive effect, but the ultimate solution to the problem of industry influence would be to remove industry from designing clinical trials altogether. We have already discussed all the ways that industry involvement in trial design undermines the reliability of data. How could we get industry out of the business of running trials? Imagine an independent body charged with prioritizing trials to answer the most important clinical questions, rather than the questions whose answers might generate the greatest profits. Once a question is chosen, centers could then compete to design and conduct the trials. This process could be, in part, supported by industry fees, as the FDA currently is. Industry could also be required to provide devices and drugs free of charge as a prerequisite to testing. The members of the committee that would design trials would need to be devoid of conflicts of interest, both past and present. A patient representative could also be included. Such a rational system would remove the grip industry currently has on the academic community.

PATTERNS OF PROMOTION AND TENURE

Let us move from the sordid influence of industry on the academic medical center to the issue of the promotion and tenure of academic faculty. Academic physicians are promoted based on their productivity, expertise, and accomplishments. What have you added to the field? Did you discover a new protein? Did you discover a new drug? Did you run a successful (likely positive) clinical trial? These are all appropriate standards. These standards reflect a central role of the academic medical center: discovery.

Discovery means generating a new and promising result. Discovery, however, is only part of what is important in science. There are two parts to research: discovery and replication. Replication is arguably the more important of the two. Replication means selecting a research study and verifying the results with a new sample or in a new setting. Replication is critical because a discovery can be a "true" discovery or a "false" discovery—random noise that only looked promising. The only way to differentiate a true discovery from a false one is to redo the experiment—ideally a few times. The need for replication is well understood. The FDA has historically required two randomized trials to show efficacy before approving a new drug. In 2014, the National Institutes of Health announced its commitment to replication by funding specific programs to make sure it happens.

Much of the debate about replication and discovery concerns preclinical research—laboratory results that test hypotheses about physiology and the mechanisms of treatments. Does this new drug attach to the opioid receptor on nerve cells? Can we improve outcomes in mice that have been engineered with a mutation in the transporter of thyroid hormone? Replication at this stage is crucial, but when it comes to reversal, replication is most important when we make the jump from theory to practice. Does this new drug decrease pain? Does the new joint last longer than the old one? Does this new implantable defibrillator save lives?

When we are trying to confirm that a treatment really works in people, we need at least two randomized trials confirming effectiveness. These trials should show benefit when you include people who look like the people who will someday use the drug. This sort of standard would prevent reversal by ensuring that a practice really works before it is used. But for this to happen, replication must be valued at least as much as discovery. Faculty need to be promoted not for discoveries that might turn out to be meaningless but for discoveries that stand the test of time—or for doing the studies that demonstrate that discoveries are valuable.

This actually runs counter to what is often the culture in the centers of discovery. No one likes a critic. There is a quiet bias that it is better to be an innovator than a critic. If you are an assistant professor trying to develop a new web-app to monitor heart rate, you are likely to get more attention than is the assistant professor who performs studies showing that this app does not improve mortality, decrease hospitalizations, or save money. In America, we like innovators. If a computer programmer makes a new game, we think it should be brought to market as soon as possible; then the public can decide. Is this game as good as *Angry Birds* or as bad as *Robotikill Fight Battles* (you never heard of it?—for good reason!)? However, as we discussed in chapter 13, medical markets are different. No one can decide what new medical technology to adopt simply based on how it looks. If you cannot judge a book by its cover, you certainly cannot judge a medical innovation by its promise.

This is why the culture of academic medicine needs to change. A recent article by Allan Brett about preoperative clearance gives a nice example of what this change should look like. Prior to elective surgery, many patients are referred to a special clinic for "clearance." This process is akin to tuning up your bike before a race. The doctors who work in these clinics try to optimize a person's health before surgery, ideally reducing complication rates. Over the years, these clinics have become dominated by guidelines, which often recommend drugs and procedures, such as cardiac stress tests, based on little or no evidence.

The preoperative clinic is now bloated with dubious practices. Dr. Brett's article took a stance against our current practice. It provided a detailed and thoughtful summary of what we do and what the evidence supports, and ultimately argued that most of the recommendations were flawed. It was a bold and inspired piece of work and required an impressive command of current evidence in the field. Yet, in the hierarchy of academic medicine, it would be classified as an "opinion piece," a status slightly higher than a case report, below observational studies, and not nearly as well respected as even a small, poorly run, before-and-after study.

Although the best work in medicine is not always a discovery, discoveries of any quality are what are lauded and valued most in the process of promotions. Replication of results, or careful, thoughtful, unbiased thinking about the results we do have, is terribly undervalued. We need to recognize and support faculty who work slowly on "opinion pieces." The process of thinking, debating, and arguing is usually more valuable, scientifically, than generating funds by running industry-sponsored trials. We need to empower the faculty at academic centers to be critics—in the best sense of the word. We need academic medicine to reflect the vibrant and contentious world that universities are supposed to be. The output should be less about what is new and potentially profitable and more about whether what we are doing really works.

We have talked about how discovery is highly valued within academia and how replication and the development of reasoned opinion is undervalued. What gets even less acclaim in academics is the actual doctoring and teaching. Although most institutions proclaim a tripartite mission of patient care, education, and discovery (usually referred to as scholarship), when it comes to promotion, discovery counts more heavily than patient care and education. If you are an excellent clinician, there is no clear path to a tenured professorship. No one takes a look at your diagnostic and therapeutic acumen and gives you credit for being the doctor to whom doctors send their families. This is not entirely inappropriate. The academic medical center exists to do more than care for patients. However, the centers would not exist if they did not provide exceptional patient care. Measuring clinical excellence is difficult. There is no canonical standard for what makes a good doctor. But, at the same time, practicing evidence-based medicine— keeping up with the latest studies and erring on the side of doing only what works—could be better assessed if we were motivated to practice this way.

USELESS RESEARCH

Here is a statement that we are uneasy about putting on paper: There is a lot of research that gets done in medicine that is useless. This statement sounds offensive and runs contrary to everything we have been taught: any search for knowledge is good and may yield great results decades hence. Each month, however, we read dozens of articles in major journals that tell us nothing new and nothing surprising.

For instance, hundreds of hours are spent studying the effects of exercise in observational data sets. Let us say: please stop. Should you exercise? Yes. Of course! Get out there and go for a walk, a swim, a bike ride. Cross-country ski in the winter and play basketball with friends in the summer. Stay hydrated, and don't kill yourself. Exercise feels good and probably improves health. And, yet, each year, hundreds of researchers perform more observational studies showing that exercise is good for you. Exercise is associated with lower rates of heart disease, and diabetes, and pancreatic cancer, and whatever. One more study on the benefits of exercise among the healthy is not needed. We have reached consensus. The people who are not exercising are not waiting for one more piece of evidence to start.

It is easy to list some of the topics that do not require more observational research. Should you eat moderately or gorge yourself? Should you eat plenty of fruits or vegetables? Is fast food bad for you? Is sleep deprivation bad? Is smoking bad? Each year, dozens of new studies prove that smoking is bad. Taxpayer money funds research to demonstrate that eating fruits and vegetables is good for you. Sadly, publishing a study saying that smoking increases your risk of pancreatic cancer is better for an academic doctor's career than working with a patient to get her to stop smoking.

There is one commonality among all this research that we put under the heading "useless." In each case, a researcher tries to link something all of us already believe is good and valuable (exercise, eating more fruits and vegetables) to specific good outcomes—or something we all think is completely unredeemable (smoking), to specific outcomes we wish to avoid (pancreatic cancer or stroke). But the link between any one factor and any one outcome found in an observational study is likely very weak. Future work may very well reverse that particular claim, but the general point will likely remain correct.

At the same time, this work diverts effort from research that could be done on the same topics that would actually provide meaningful information. For instance, exercise is great, but there are very few randomized trials showing that a specific exercise recommendation can help a specific group of patients. One of these rare gems is a trial showing that weight-lifting actually improves lymphedema symptoms for women who have had a lymph node dissection as part of the treatment for their breast cancer. What type of exercise program is best for patients with arthritis? Emphysema? These are questions best tested in randomized trials, and the valuable answers could be confidently deployed in medical practice.

A general recommendation about how to transform useless research into useful research is to perform trials of specific interventions on specific populations. Instead of an observational study showing that smoking slows healing after wrist injuries, how about a study showing whether a particular smoking cessation strategy improves survival among patients with diabetes? Simply demonstrating—over and over again in observational studies—that smoking is bad for you is like the movie *Groundhog Day* without Bill Murray and Andie MacDowell ever falling in love.

Yes, replication is important, but flogging a dead horse is not. These topics are chosen over and over because it is easy to publish this work (and get press coverage of it). These studies, however, do not push us forward as a profession.

How does this relate to reversal? Useless research often produces poorly founded conclusions that are then acted upon. Only later do we learn that our interventions were ineffective. Performing the types of studies we suggest might reveal therapies that run counter to what we would have guessed. We told you that a gem of a study found that weight-lifting improves symptoms of lymphedema. This was an example of reversal (see study 126 in the appendix). For years, doctors told women not to lift weights after their lymph nodes had been removed, for fear it would worsen the condition.

When you actually begin to test ways to implement what you think you know, you start to learn interesting things.

AN EXCELLENT PHYSICIAN

For all the reasons presented in this chapter, we have to do better to define what makes an excellent physician. An excellent doctor is not the one who studies whether eating strawberries in moderation is good for you. He should not be on the nightly news or necessarily promoted at his university, especially while the doctor who will hold your hand while she tells you the test results that no one wished for is penalized for not being academically productive.

The ideal academic doctor is someone who spends a modest portion of his time caring for patients and the balance teaching, reading, thinking, and conducting research—research aimed at discovery or replication of potentially important findings. The ideal doctor is not someone who spends four months at conferences, collects honoraria, and works as a tireless advocate for industry. The best publications, research or thought pieces, are those that engage the medical community and prompt it to think about how to best care for people. They are not the next industry-sponsored, uncontrolled device trial. The best professor is someone who inspires her students to become better doctors. She is not the one who gives students a gift authorship on a paper showing that exercise improves blood flow. A productive faculty member is not the one who brings in $2 million from GlaxoSmithKline, but the one who brings wisdom and compassion to the bedside, to his students, and to his trainees and develops thoughtful research questions during his clinical work. Medical reversal is, in part, the price we pay because what we value in the academic medical center has become skewed.

A little reform might go a long way toward making sure the goals of academic medical centers are what we believe them to be: to promote human health. Interventions to realign these goals must be studied to determine whether the modified goals really do produce better patient care and more robust discoveries. If they do, they should be widely adopted. If they do not, we should go back to the drawing board so that we do not reform our medical centers only to have to reverse ourselves in the future.

16
REFORMING THE SYSTEM

:: THE BURDEN OF PROOF AND NUDGING
OUR WAY PAST REVERSAL

MEDICAL REVERSALS ARE EVERYWHERE. They are rooted in our tendency to accept new practices without really knowing that they work. So far in this part of the book, we have suggested that reforming medical education and academic medicine could lessen the prevalence of reversal. We have also listened to our own sermon: we have tried to caution that most of our reforms are not ready for prime time and should be subject to pilot programs and testing in randomized trials. In this chapter, we introduce two more proposals. Both are ambitious and both take aim at the foundation of medical reversal. One requires a new ethic among drug and device developers, and the other calls patients and doctors to commit themselves to clinical trials.

THE BURDEN OF PROOF

Semper necessitas probandi incumbit ei qui agit. The necessity of proof always lies with him who lays the charges. This legal principle, if applied to medical innovation, would go a long way toward curbing reversal.

The principle of burden of proof means that for a given claim, one side has the burden of proof—the responsibility to show that its statement is true—while the opposing side has the benefit of assumption. If the first side is unable to prove its claim, the other side is assumed to be correct. An example makes the principle clear. Imagine that a PhD student in biology is doing a dissertation on the reptiles of the Nicaraguan rain forest. He returns from a field expedition and claims that he discovered a new species of snake. The snake he found is longer than a boa constrictor, spends most of its life under water, has the ability to alter its colors (like a chameleon), and has a sharp barb at the end of its tail. The question is, Does this hitherto undiscovered snake exist? The obligation to produce evidence falls upon the graduate student. He could show a picture of the snake. He could produce a molted skin. He could bring a specimen, dead or (terrifyingly) alive. These pieces of evidence would rank on a scale of lesser to nearly certain proof.

In contrast, a skeptic of the "new snake" theory has no burden of proof. How can someone prove that a snake does not exist? One might produce an array of circumstantial evidence. Among all graduate students who claim to have discovered a new species of snake, what percentage is correct? Moreover, the discovery rate has surely changed over time. We might guess that in the 19th century, perhaps 20 percent of "new discoveries" were truly new, but by 2015, this number has surely fallen, perhaps as low as 1 percent. The skeptic might also show how a previously described snake, indigenous to Nicaragua, could be mistaken for this "new snake." In the right light and against the right tree, could this have been a Central American tree boa? But a skeptic can never "prove" that the snake does not exist. The burden of proof, in cases of newly discovered species, must be on the discoverer.

The burden-of-proof principle is not just a legal principle, but a fundamental principle of logical assertions. Depending on the claim, one party has the obligation to prove it is true. If a friend says he can drive from Chicago to Washington, D.C., in five hours, you can be skeptical, knowing the drive takes you twice as long, but you cannot disprove the claim. It's up to your friend to prove his own claim.

In law, the burden of proof is an accepted concept. For murder cases, the burden rests on the prosecutor to prove that the defendant committed the crime. It is not up to the accused to prove his innocence. For malpractice claims, the plaintiff has to show the doctor was at fault. The doctor's actions must have *directly* contributed to *damage* (some harm a patient experiences) and must have constituted *dereliction* of the doctor's *duty*. Proving these "4 Ds" is the plaintiff's burden of proof.

Although its application seems sensible, the concept of the burden of proof is not really considered when we think about medical innovation. Every doctor has been part of a conversation that goes something like this.

DR. SMITH: "There is no evidence that what you are suggesting works."

DR. JONES: "True, but there is no evidence that it does not work, is there?"

In fact, there is a saying in medicine that captures the extent to which this debate is alive: "*The absence of evidence is not evidence of absence.*" Not having proof that a treatment works is not proof that it does not work. In the day-to-day care of patients, when the evidence base for what needs to be done is often thin, this statement might, on occasion, make sense (more on this in chapter 18). However, it should not be applied to new drugs or devices.

The burden of proof has a long-standing tradition in medicine with varying standards and requirements, but its modern incarnation began with a major expansion of the FDA's power in the approval of new medications. For the first half of the 20th century, the U.S. Food and Drug Administration was charged with ensuring the safety of drugs. Whether or not a drug actually did what was advertised was not a requirement for approval. Then in 1962, with the passage of the Kefauver-Harris Amendment, the agency was given the additional task of ensuring the efficacy of drugs. Since that time, a drug developer has to show some evidence that the new drug actually does what it is purported to do. Of course, as we discussed in chapter 12, there are many ways that this requirement has been eroded. The accelerated-approval pathway allows drugs to come to market if they improve surrogate end points that are "reasonably likely to predict" true efficacy. In several dramatic cases, like that of bevacizumab in breast cancer (chapter 3), this policy has allowed drugs to reach the market that ultimately had no value (and sometimes did harm).

Medicine's experience with device development perfectly illustrates the lack of a clear standard of burden of proof. Many medical devices have been approved for use with little evidence that they work—the maker was not forced to prove that the product would work. A wonderful (and disturbing) example is the inferior-vena-cava filter used to treat pulmonary embolism. Pulmonary embolism occurs when blood clots form, usually in the legs, often after a period of immobility (after surgery, a long car ride, or a flight from Istanbul) and then embolize ("travel") to the lungs. When these clots lodge in the lungs' circulation, they can be deadly. The inferior-vena-cava (IVC) filter is one of those ingenious inventions that seems like it should work. It is a small metallic basket, placed in the large vessel between the legs and the lungs, that is intended to catch a blood clot before it reaches the lungs. This device has been widely used for decades. We have both prescribed IVC filters for patients (admittedly, largely before we investigated the device). However, to date, there is no evidence that this basket actually improves any patient outcomes. There is clear evidence that having the basket implanted in your body causes harms—an increase in leg pain, swelling, and the risk of recurrent blood clots in the legs. The device gained approval through an FDA pathway (510k) that demands neither safety nor efficacy data.

The debate around the use of the IVC filter perfectly illustrates why we need to clarify the burden of proof in medical innovation. On the one side are skeptics who (rightly) argue that there is no good evidence that the IVC filter works and that its use should be restricted to randomized trials testing its benefit. On the other side are believers who argue that the IVC filter has certainly not been resoundingly disproved and may work. "Why not use it?" they ask. In this debate the believers are winning, and the device is implanted hundreds of times each day in America.

Much of medicine happens here, in the no-man's-land in which there is little evidence that a treatment helps and often evidence that it may do harm. We believe it is time to formalize the burden-of-proof principle and set a high bar in medicine by requiring developers to clearly prove that an innovation works prior to its adoption. Currently (you have heard this before), new interventions are often debuted and accepted into practice before they have been shown to benefit patients in robust clinical trials. This is not done for malicious reasons but because the therapies make sense and all involved (developers, doctors, patients) hope that they will work. Years may then pass before the treatment is put to the test in large, well-done randomized trials. These trials, when they are finally completed, not infrequently show that the treatment is ineffective. In America today, it is not the innovators and manufacturers who are carrying the burden of proof to design, pay for, and run these trials. Instead, it is third parties funding creative (and brave) researchers who are willing to challenge medical standards years after the introduction of these widely used (and often highly profitable) therapies. This must change. The burden of proof that an intervention works must be borne by those who develop a new therapy and by the practitioners who prescribe it (both of whom are likely to profit from it).

:: THREE ARGUMENTS FOR THE BURDEN OF PROOF

We believe in a careful adherence to the burden-of-proof principle for three reasons. The first, alluded to above, is that placing the burden of proof on the developers of the therapies is the most practical approach. It is easier and safer to prove that a treatment works before deploying it widely, than to prove that the therapy does not work (or does harm) after it is widely available. Although it may be easier to prove that placing coronary-artery stents does not benefit people with stable coronary-artery disease than it is to prove that a species of snake does not exist, such proof is predictably followed by caveat seekers. "Sure you proved stents do not work in *that* population," they say, "but how about in older people, or people with diabetes, or people with higher cholesterol levels?" The appropriate response, and one that must be the new normal, is to begin with the proof that the intervention is truly and unquestionably effective for the indication it is claimed to help.

The second reason to endorse a strong burden of proof is that so few medical innovations actually are successful. Among all medical innovations, what percent are likely to work? You might think back to chapter 7 and say about half of them. That is the figure we arrived at from our work and that of the *British Medical Journal Clinical Evidence* project (figure 7.2). However, it is worth remembering that we were asking what proportion of innovations that are already widely accepted are effective. Now we are asking, instead, what proportion of all medical innovations are likely to work. Half is probably an overestimate. The number is likely to be quite low. Of 100 drugs that are conceived, at most 1 successfully becomes a commercial product and an even smaller proportion are resoundingly effective. This would give a rate of less than 1 percent. Moreover, as we have seen, no observational studies (no matter how many) or mechanistic logic is sufficient to prove that a treatment will work. Recently a drug that by all measures should have been better than placebo in the treatment of liver cancer was found not to work. The authors of the study wrote, "Despite the strong scientific rationale [they go on to cite nine references] and preclinical data [four references!] [the experimental drug] plus [the] best supportive care failed to improve survival over placebo and the best supportive care." In short, the probability that a therapeutic intervention actually works is very, very low—despite abundant "promising" and "encouraging" studies.

Third, our argument for a strong burden of proof rests on the medical principle of *primum non nocere*—first, do no harm. By all means, a doctor's goal should be to recommend treatments that benefit his patients. But if he cannot do that—if he cannot offer an intervention that has been tested and proved, then, at a minimum, he must do no harm. Better not to "give it a shot" and cause problems. Instead, perhaps the best thing to do is to provide support and comfort to the patient. From a historical standpoint, this principle would have served doctors well. Just think of bloodletting, trephination,* and arsenic therapy for syphilis. In the modern world, as in the past, doctors and patients often think that *giving it a shot* is preferable. But, if you think that, refer back to chapter 7.

:: BEHAVIORAL CHANGES

Where would adoption of this standard of burden of proof require behaviors to change the most? The sites of greatest change would be in regulatory agencies and in doctors' offices. First, because doctors can only prescribe and recommend drugs and devices that are approved, we suggest that all approvals by the regulatory agencies must be based on clear evidence of safety and efficacy. Furthermore, the efficacy of a new treatment must be demonstrated to be at least equivalent to accepted and proven treatment options combined with the best medical care. A developer cannot test a marginal drug in a Third World country with no other care, show a benefit over placebo, and try to apply that result to the U.S. market, where patients would be getting other approved drugs and the best supportive care.[†] Clearly, placing the burden of proof on drug and device developers

---

* Trephination is the act of boring holes into a patient's skull for medical benefit. Although there are times this is medically indicated in the 21st century, there is a long history of using trephination for misguided reasons, such as to allow bad humors to escape.

† A good example of this involved afatinib, a drug for lung cancer, which was tested in less-developed countries against a regimen inferior to the global standard of care.

and holding the regulatory approval process to exacting standards by which to evaluate the data provided are important steps in decreasing reversal. It is nothing more than asking the FDA to fulfill the charge of the agency: ensure safety and efficacy prior to approval.

Second, doctors themselves will need to change the way they practice. Just because the FDA approves a drug or device does not mean it automatically enters widespread usage; this requires that doctors recommend it. Here too, adopting the burden of proof would require new practices. Before a doctor recommends a treatment to a patient, she should ask herself whether there is good evidence that it works. At a minimum, if there is not strong evidence of efficacy, that information should be shared with patients. More radically, if the evidence is not there, the doctor should not offer the intervention.

These behavioral changes will not be easy—especially for regulatory agencies. For the past 20 years, first with accelerated approval and now with the FDA's "breakthrough designation," more and more pills can reach the marketplace without good evidence that they improve the end points important to patients.* When one considers not just pills but devices and surgeries, regulatory agencies have often not insisted that inventors provide good evidence that their inventions work prior to their debut. It is worth noting that we are not alone in insisting on this provision of proof. When the Institute of Medicine considered the FDA's device-approval process, it called for the most permissive pathway (called 510k) to be eliminated. It is time that we, as a society, make sure we get things right in medicine while the horse is still in the barn. One of the lessons of medical reversal is that horses are very difficult to rein in once they are loose.

NUDGING OUR WAY FORWARD

If the medical field accepts this new ethic and agrees that the burden of proving that a new treatment is effective should be placed on developers

---

* In 2012 the FDA adopted the Breakthrough Therapy Designation. To achieve this designation, a drug must be intended "to treat a serious or life threatening disease or condition and have preliminary clinical evidence indicat[ing] that [it] may demonstrate substantial improvement over existing therapies on one or more clinically significant endpoints, such as substantial treatment effects observed early in clinical development." Drugs designated as breakthrough therapy receive expedited review.

and upheld by regulators and prescribers, we will need to vastly increase the number of therapies being tested in randomized controlled trials. How do we accomplish this?

Frequently at a restaurant, while you wait for your food (or your server), you are served complimentary bread, or chips and salsa. Is this a beneficial practice for the restaurant? Recently the Freakonomics Radio Podcast dedicated an episode to this question. Many interested parties debated whether an *amuse-bouche* increased or decreased a restaurant's revenue. One argument went that a free appetizer would fill people up, lead to the ordering of less food or fewer desserts, and thus decrease revenue. Another argument was that yes, free bread does those things, but in doing so it makes people leave sooner, freeing up the table for another seating. Even though the restaurant moves fewer desserts, there is more table traffic and, in the end, the restaurant makes more money. You could argue about this forever (and, in fact, the discussion on this podcast did become a bit inane), or you could do a randomized controlled trial. But what would you randomize? Would it be each table? In that case, the worry is that if a control table sees that another table is getting free bread, the customers at the control table may feel put out. Perhaps you could randomize several restaurants? How about a nationwide study in which 200 restaurants that do not serve free bread are randomized to offering it or not and sales are followed. In just a few weeks, we would have an answer that might end up changing restaurant practices globally. Why have we not seen this study? The problem: how do you get all of those restaurants to participate?

Sure, this example is silly, but the question of how to get restaurants enrolled is an important one. How do you increase participation in trials? In medicine there are countless important questions that small, simple trials could easily answer. The barrier is getting people to enter the trial. Consider the story of pediatric versus adult cancers. For most of the 1990s, pediatricians developed a rich and comprehensive network so that nearly all children with cancer were enrolled in some form of clinical trial. Much of their success—large improvements in survival for their patients—is attributed to the push for clinical trials. In contrast, to date, less than 10 percent of adult cancer patients participate in clinical trials, and, arguably, adult care has lagged behind. Of course, we cannot really compare improvements in adult and pediatric cancer care—they are apples and oranges. That being said, the comparison is hypothesis-generating. Would medicine be better if a larger proportion of patients were enrolled in clinical trials? and if so, how might we entice (or nudge) these subjects into trials?

Richard Thaler, a professor of behavioral science and economics, and Cass Sunstein, a professor of law, introduced the nudge principle in their book *Nudge: Improving Decisions about Health, Wealth, and Happiness*. This principle might suggest the way to increase enrollment in clinical trials. The nudge principle is simple: if you want people to do something, make that action the default option while still letting them opt out if they want to. For years, activists tried everything to improve the percentage of people who volunteered to be organ donors. The simple solution is to change the question from "Do you want to donate?" to "Do you not want to donate?" For many things—from retirement savings accounts to healthy choices in the school lunch line—simply changing the default, while giving people the freedom to opt out, dramatically increases the desired behavior.

How would the nudge principle work in medicine? Consider, as an example, the treatment of pneumonia. There are numerous potential treatments, and nobody really knows which is better. What if we said to the next 1,000 pneumonia patients, "There are many different ways to treat this infection. All of them work, but we do not know which is best. To study this, we are going to randomly pick one of these effective treatments for you, unless you want to opt out." Most people would probably say, "Sure, that's fine." We doubt that many people have an allegiance to moxifloxacin over ceftriaxone. What if every patient who sought care in the hospital contributed not just to a single trial, but to multiple studies?

The number of questions that could be easily and quickly studied in this way is exciting. The questions do not need to be profound ones. Is it better to let the average hospitalized patient sleep through the night, or should we wake her to measure her blood pressure (as we presently do). With enough patients, you could have a definitive trial done in a month. One of the most common reasons for admission to the hospital is syncope, the transient loss of consciousness and postural tone—in lay terms, fainting. Often, a patient's history alone reveals the diagnosis, but sometimes the cause is more enigmatic. Presently we spend a lot of time and energy (and money) evaluating these patients. Does every person really need every test? A few randomized trials of a thousand people could optimize our approach to syncope.

The beauty of the nudge principle is that nobody's choice is being taken away. In 2015, you can choose to participate in a trial, or not. In 2020, the choice would still be yours. All we propose is to change the default, and the usual patient's response goes from No thanks to Sure, why not. This change would have to be accompanied by the creation of a robust clinical-trials enterprise able to design studies and conduct them, at low cost, with fewer barriers across diverse settings. For most clinical questions, those for which we really do not know the answer, there should be no barriers to additional trials. If a physician has a patient with a problem for which there are no treatments supported by a robust evidence base, that physician should be able to begin a trial, quickly and easily. Obviously, the busy practicing clinician cannot do this alone. The infrastructure needs to be created.

There will be reasonable opposition to using the nudge principle to increase trial enrollment. Groups that have historically been marginalized may feel that being enrolled in trials is exploitative. Although we would argue, as Thaler and Sunstein do, that the choice to not participate is still present and that the default option is merely switched, patients' ability to opt out of trials would have to be made very clear to them so there is no hint of coercion. Great care would have to be taken to make sure the therapies being offered in a trial really are truly considered equivalent. The reality is that few of us are likely to feel strongly about the decision; most of us would be indifferent about which of two putatively equivalent treatments we would receive.

Another real concern is, Who designs these studies? We know that the pharmaceutical and device industries tend to design trials with their interests in mind. We endorse the nudge principle only for trials designed and conducted by teams who have no conflicts of interest. The nudge principle is a tool. If used correctly, it could do a lot of good; if used improperly, it could accelerate harm.

Finally, the nudge principle should be instituted alongside a broader commitment to conduct clinical trials for less money. Right now, researchers estimate that it costs $5,000 to $20,000 per patient per trial just to handle enrollment and data management. Like most costs in health care, this is absurd. Researchers know that being in a trial does not increase the cost of your medical care and that the cost of handling the data from that trial must be decreased. There are many ways of achieving this. One potential solution is the development of registry-based randomized trials. These are trials conducted within existing observational studies that would therefore decrease costs of patient recruitment. In one such study, the cost to randomize each patient fell to $50.

MEDICAL CARE IN AN ERA OF A HIGH BURDEN OF PROOF AND STREAMLINED CLINICAL TRIALS

Instituting a clear requirement of the burden of proof in medical innovation and using the nudge principle to increase enrollment in clinical trials are closely related and interdependent recommendations. Setting the evidentiary bar higher for the adoption of new therapies risks slowing down medical innovation. Reforming how we recruit people into trials would not only avoid this negative consequence but actually improve the present situation. If innovations are tested quickly, we can assure that an innovation that is adopted is really a beneficial one.

Patient care would look different in a world with a high burden of proof and a streamlined system of trial recruitment. There might actually be fewer options for treatment, but this would not be a bad thing. The options that would no longer exist would be the ones that do not work (or actually cause harm). Currently, patients who exhaust proven remedies are offered a menu of unproven treatments. In the world we envision, these patients would not be treated with guesses but would have a range of clinical trials to choose from. They would be given novel treatments, but in a setting that protects their health. The safest way to receive a new drug is in a trial with a control arm. The randomized-controlled-trial design provides a built-in safeguard—trials are stopped if the treatment turns out to be harmful (remember the CAST study from chapter 1). When patients are treated with unproven medicines outside trials, there is no safety net.

::

There are more unanswered questions in medicine than we could ever count. Each day patients and doctors must make choices. The byproduct of this situation is that many decisions turn out to be wrong and many accepted medical practices turn out to be major missteps. We need a way forward that assures that we get it right more often. We propose reforms that we believe would go a long way toward curbing reversal: medical innovations should be subject to higher regulatory and professional standards that are based on adoption of the concept of the burden of proof and a commitment to answering relevant clinical questions, facilitated through use of the nudge principle. The specific solutions we suggest should be evaluated. Clever trials can assess whether the nudge principle improves patient outcomes or whether the trials that get done are trivial and accomplish little. We believe these proposals are logical and compelling and that it is time to put them to the test.

17 / HOW NOT TO BECOME A VICTIM OF REVERSAL

THE STRUCTURE AND CULTURE of the medical field makes it likely that you will be offered therapies that are unproven. Some of these therapies will eventually be reversed. In this chapter we propose a way to approach your medical care that minimizes the risk that you will receive a therapy today that will be found to be ineffective or harmful tomorrow. By taking a smart approach to your care and forming a productive alliance with your doctor, you can (mostly) assure yourself excellent, evidence-based, care. We say "mostly" because, as we have outlined, there are strong forces behind the epidemic of reversal. Financial incentives, a confidence in mechanistic science, and a medical literature filled with studies designed and run by the companies that stand to profit from the outcome—all of these promote faulty therapies. At times, even we, as physicians, have been tricked. During our careers we have written prescriptions for estrogen-replacement therapy, fenofibrate, and other interventions that were based on flawed evidence but good stories.

Your basic goal as a patient is easily stated: you need to be confident that every medical intervention you accept has been shown, in robust studies, to improve the outcome in which you are most interested. If no such treatment exists (not an uncommon scenario, even in 21st-century medicine), you should be aware that the effectiveness of any therapy you consider is based more on conjecture and hope than on science. Sometimes accepting such therapies is reasonable, but that acceptance should be a highly informed decision.

There is much working against you, coming from both sides of the doctor-patient relationship, in achieving this goal. From the patient side of the equation, there is what has been called "white-coat silence." This term is analogous to white-coat hypertension, a phenomenon in which people who have normal blood pressures become hypertensive when they come to the doctor. White-coat silence occurs when a usually informed, confident, and empowered person walks into a doctor's office and fails to ask the important questions. The causes of this phenomenon are likely legion and, to a great extent, unknown, but it is real. But simply asking questions is not everything. It takes skill to ask the right questions about decisions that you do not know much about. How is a patient just diagnosed with angina supposed to know what medications should be prescribed for him?

On the doctor's side, the two challenges are time and knowledge. Patients returning to Adam's practice are scheduled in 20-minute intervals to allow (or force) him to see 12 patients in a four-hour session. This, of course, ignores the one or two people who are added during each session with urgent issues. Vinayak often finds himself having to see two patients at once—one admitted in the hospital and another arriving at the clinic. In accordance with Murphy's Law, this usually happens right when a third patient calls. For these reasons, it is hard to get a harried doctor to sit back and reconsider decisions that he has made. Even more of a challenge is that many physicians do not have the knowledge at hand to answer the questions you should ask. A busy doctor often gets information about therapeutics from guidelines and pharmaceutical detailers rather than the weekly medical journals. Even for those who do religiously consume the *New England Journal of Medicine* and the *Journal of the American Medical Association*, it has become harder and harder to identify the interventions that really make a difference. The design and reporting of trials is frequently (and in some cases purposely) complicated in an effort to make drugs look more effective than they are.

So, where do we start? We start by asking the right questions. Patients often gravitate toward the nuts and bolts of a recommendation. How does it work? What are the side effects? Does my insurance cover it? These are great questions—but are for a later time. Vertebroplasty, discussed in chapter 1, came with a great story. It also had few side effects and was covered by most insurance plans. The real question should have been, Does it work?

STEP 1. WHAT END POINTS MATTER?

When presented with a medical recommendation, start with a bit of soul-searching. What end points matter to you? We discussed many of these issues in chapter 3 when we talked about surrogate end points. Anything measurable can be an end point, but do not be fooled; not all end points are equal. If we are perfectly honest, only two end points matter: morbidity and mortality. Morbidity: will this treatment relieve my symptoms, or free me from or prevent future disability? Mortality: will this treatment make me live longer?

When a doctor suggests a treatment, take a second to think about what end points matter to you. This really gets back to surrogate end points, those end points that are easy to measure, which generally track with more important clinical end points but are, in themselves, meaningless. We covered these in detail in chapter 3. Let us imagine that you are meeting with your doctor to initiate treatment for recently diagnosed diabetes. You feel well; in fact you did not even suspect there was anything wrong with you until a blood test showed that you had elevated blood sugars. Your doctor suggests a medicine and says that this medication will effectively lower your blood sugar and hemoglobin A1c (HbA1c), the number that we use to monitor the average blood sugar. The questions to ask at this point are these: Why do we treat diabetes? What are the end points we are trying to avoid? The responses to these questions serve as the launching point for the rest of the discussion.

We treat diabetes not to get better blood-sugar numbers but because lowering blood sugars leads to fewer symptoms (frequent urination, insatiable thirst) and, ideally, avoids the late complications of the disease: blindness, nerve injury, kidney failure, heart attacks, strokes, and death. The specifics are important because not all treatments that lower blood sugar lessen the real burden of the disease—recall Thomas Galbraith back in chapter 3.

Sometimes the disconnect between the real, important outcomes and the stand-in, the surrogate outcome, can be truly disconcerting. A patient with bladder cancer that has spread to his liver and lung might be offered a treatment that has been proved to shrink tumors. This is not an important outcome. The patient may not feel the tumors. What matters is whether the drug helps the person to live as long as possible with the fewest symptoms. There are plenty of examples of treatments that shrink tumors but do not improve the end points you care about.

Now you could try to take this a step further and research the relationship between the surrogate and the end point you care about. How reliable is bone density as a marker of future hip fracture? How good is carotid-artery intimal thickness at predicting heart attacks? Be careful. Surrogates mislead frequently, and no one has perfectly figured out the rhyme or reason to it.

STEP 2. WHAT TYPE OF STUDIES SHOWS THAT THE TREATMENT IMPROVES THE END POINTS THAT MATTER?

If you are lucky enough to find that there is evidence that the treatment you have been offered affects the end point you are interested in, you next must determine whether this is reliable evidence. We hope our earlier discussions have convinced you that faulty evidence is not really any better than no evidence at all. If the evidence is one doctor's experience or an observational study—you should doubt it. You would like the evidence to come from a randomized trial done at hospitals across the country.

But then you should also ask, How good is that randomized trial? This is a question that attentive doctors spend a lot of time thinking about but one that will be very hard for you, as a patient, to answer on your own. Not all randomized controlled trials are created equal and not every trial applies to every patient. Are the patients in the trial like you? Same age? Same problems? Same fitness? Same country? Who paid for this trial? Was it a government-sponsored trial that was trying to discover the truth or an industry-sponsored one that was trying to sell a drug?

Before going on to Step 3, it is time to pause and consider what you have been offered. If the treatment suggested has not been proved, in a well-done randomized trial, to benefit the outcome in which you are interested, you need to ask about alternative treatments. We are fortunate to live at a time when there are usually alternatives. Many of the alternatives are older, less expensive, well-proven treatments. They may not be the hottest new drug with an impressive advertising campaign, but they may be more effective. Note the "may be." It goes without saying that you should ask the same questions about the alternative treatments.

It may be hard to get these alternatives. Doctors will sometimes gloss over them. They have reasons for their recommendations, and there are reasons why the alternatives are just that, alternatives—but this is your decision. Get a couple of options, write them down, and ask the right questions. A key question at this point is, What happens if we do nothing? In doctorspeak, this means, What is the natural history of the disease? Lots of doctors do not know the answer to this question for diseases they treat all the time. Why? Well, because it is so rare that we do nothing. For some conditions, the natural history is just to get better (or not to get worse). That is the case for most musculoskeletal injuries and, as the medical profession has learned recently, for some early-stage, caught-only-by-screening, cancers. For some conditions, the natural history is death. Natural history can be based on old data, data for patients with severe versions of illness, or data from a few cases. Do these data apply today, to you?

STEP 3. HOW MUCH WILL THIS TREATMENT HELP?

If you are lucky and have been offered a treatment that addresses the end points you care about and has been proved in a well-done, randomized controlled trial, the answer to this question will help you decide whether the therapy is worth it. It will help you weigh risks and benefits. You need to ask your doctor the "number needed to treat." How many people like me need to get this therapy, for what period of time, for one person to benefit from it? The size of this number will always surprise you. Our best therapies that are meant to prolong life (outside the realm of cancer care) require us to treat 20 to 50 patients to provide benefit to one. Treating patients with cholesterol-lowering statin drugs after an MI may be gospel in medicine, but you need to treat 20 people for five years to save one life. The numbers are even greater for preventive interventions. Few people question colon-cancer screening, but it takes doing endoscopy on 191 people and following them for 11 years to prevent one case of colon cancer. You will need to consider this likelihood of benefit compared to side effects, costs, and the hassle of the therapy to decide whether this treatment is right for you.

STEP 4. MAKING THE DECISION

If you have been offered a treatment that is proved to affect end points you care about, you can decide whether you want it. You have considered the "number needed to treat." Now ask those questions that you wanted to ask from the start. How does it work? What are the side effects? Does my insurance cover it?

If the only therapy for a problem is an unproven one, your decision whether to accept it depends on your state of health. If you are lucky enough not to have a medical problem and you feel well, the decision is easy. In this case, the unproven treatment that you are being offered is to prevent you from becoming ill. To quote Nancy Reagan, "Just say no." The likelihood that such a treatment will improve the things that matter is very low. The list of medical practices that improve outcomes among healthy individuals is a very short one.* If you are sick or suffering, the decision is harder. The treatment you are being offered may help, but it also may not. This is true no matter how convincing the surrogate end points are, how convincing the explanation of how the treatment should work is, or how well produced the advertisements are. It is in your best interest (as well as your doctor's) to understand that you are accepting the treatment knowing that there is a fairly good possibility it will not work. Remember that the majority of people do not even benefit from the treatments that every doctor agrees are indicated.†

Consider three patients. The first is a patient with elevated bad cholesterol and low good cholesterol. In 2006 she was 55 years old and had had diabetes for five years. Her doctor prescribed niacin. There were trials showing that it raised good cholesterol and lowered bad cholesterol. The mechanism of action is elegant. The drug acts in several parts of the cholesterol pathway. Moreover, the patient tolerated the drug well, without flushing, the most common side effect. Finally, the drug was FDA-approved and was covered by the patient's insurance. However, there were no studies that proved the drug improved clinical end points—cardiovascular outcomes

---

* Vaccinations, both childhood and adult, are on this list.
† Consider the cholesterol-lowering statin medicine after a heart attack discussed above: 19 out of 20 patients given this well-proven medicine will not have their life saved by it.

and death. The patient took the medication for years before it became clear that niacin does not improve these outcomes.

The second patient is a 44-year-old man, an avid runner. On a morning jog he tripped and fell, rupturing his hamstring. Traditionally this injury was treated with rest and physical therapy. Some patients did well; others had persistent pain and disability. His doctor, knowing how important running was to this man, referred him to an orthopedic surgeon who recommended surgical repair. The studies that support this intervention were poorly designed: they compared the outcomes of patients who were offered (and chose to have) surgery with those who were not (or did not). The rationale behind the procedure was logical; the surgeon would reattach the hamstring to where it had been for the previous 44 years. The patient, wanting to know he had done everything to improve his chances, chose to have the surgery. After six weeks of immobility and six weeks of therapy, he is back to his baseline performance. Of course, we do not know whether the surgery made the difference, but the runner does not care.

The third is perhaps the most challenging case. A 72-year-old man with thyroid cancer that has spread to his lungs begins to get symptoms from his cancer. He feels "tightness" in his neck and shortness of breath. Without a doubt, he has a serious condition that, unfortunately, will eventually lead to his demise. A new medication comes on the market (vandetanib) expressly for his cancer. A lot of things make the drug attractive. For starters, it is a pill (not an intravenous treatment) that you only have to take once a day. But there are significant downsides. The side effects are so bad that about one-third of patients cannot tolerate the starting dose, and 12 percent end up having to stop taking it altogether. These numbers are based upon the patients who are fit enough to participate in a randomized trial that studied the drug. For patients outside of trials, cancer drugs often have worse side effects. Vandetanib was approved by the FDA because it slows the growth of the tumor, but it did not show any improvement in survival. (Remember bevacizumab in chapter 3.) What does all this mean? It makes for a very tough decision. The patient, with his doctor, has to balance the symptoms he is currently having against any side effects he might develop if he takes the drug, while knowing that the drug may not make him live a single day longer.

Decision making without data is hard. It is also, often, necessary.

STEP 5. FIND SOMEONE WITH WHOM YOU CAN WORK

You and your doctor will need to work together to figure out what is the right treatment for you. When there are data, they might require you to ask questions that will require some legwork on your doctor's part. When there are no data, you will need honest advice from someone you trust. It is helpful to get a sense of the doctor's philosophy and make sure it matches your own. We all want good care, but some may want a "less is more" approach, while others prefer an aggressive, "leave no stone unturned," approach. If it is true that no one can really change, do not expect your doctor's philosophy to change completely to suit your own.

One thing that you should expect from any doctor is a willingness to answer your questions. In the hurried pace of medicine today, this may seem a lot to ask. It is not. What follow are a few suggestions about how to get the most out of your exchange with your doctor. Some of these questions and statements come from our patients and have helped them get the best care out of us; others are things we wish our patients would ask more often.

:: USE THE DOCTOR'S EXPERIENCE

Yes, your doctor has had a lot of training, but what makes the consultation valuable is that she has cared for many people having the experience that you are having for the first time. When a therapy is offered, take advantage of this. "How long have you been using this treatment?" "Before this drug/surgery was available, what were you doing, and why is this better?" "Have you read any studies that would make you doubt this treatment?"

:: USE THE DOCTOR'S EXPERTISE

If you could read and understand all the studies of all the treatments you are being offered, you would not need a doctor. Asking your doctor to explain the data can be challenging, but to make the decisions as we outlined above, you need to. Ask to see the articles that your doctor is referencing. The abstracts of articles are usually easy to understand and can open the door to asking further questions. Make it clear that you are not second-guessing. Doctors are more impressed than put off when we hear patients say,

> "I don't mean to be a problem, but this is important to me and I just want to make sure I am going to be comfortable with what I choose."
> "I trust your judgment, but I want to make sure this is right for me."

"I understand that you might not have time for this now. When is a good
time that I can come back? Or can I ask you more questions by phone
or email?"

:: AIM HIGH IN STEERING

This is probably the only phrase we still remember from driver's ed.
Sometimes the decisions that lie further ahead can inform the decisions
at hand. "If this treatment does not help, what will we do next?" "Why are
you suggesting the treatments in this order rather than the reverse?" These
questions are not only for making decisions about therapy; they apply
when considering diagnostic tests and evaluations. "If this test is negative,
what do we do?" ("Are we done?" "Will we have ruled out the disease?" If
not, "Should we start with a different test?") "If the test is positive, what will
we do?" "Is there a proven treatment?" (If there is not, do you really want to
know about the diagnosis?) "If the test is nondiagnostic, what will we do?"
"How likely is it to be nondiagnostic?"

PARTICIPATE IN RANDOMIZED TRIALS, CONDUCTED BY IMPARTIAL SPONSORS

We end with a final plea. There are clinical trials in which you should participate. We cannot endorse any or every clinical trial because, frankly,
there are some bad studies out there. If you have cancer and are interested
in a phase 1 trial, you should know that the trial is overwhelmingly unlikely
to benefit you. Your motivation should be pure altruism. If you have any
condition and are considering a study without a control arm, you have to
probe the motivation of the investigator and ask whether the trial will provide useful information—no matter how excited you are to try something
new. When considering randomized trials, remember that some industry-
sponsored studies have flawed designs or do not ask the best clinical question. On the other hand, do sign up for any randomized trial fully conducted and paid for by impartial sponsors. The National Institutes of Health,
the Veterans Administration—these are groups that conduct trials only
to answer important clinical questions. Furthermore, you would be in a
randomized trial. These are trials where there is true equipoise—we do
not know which treatment is better. Not only is your treatment conducted
with the safety of a treatment arm and a control arm; you guarantee yourself safe and effective treatment, but in addition, your care will help other

patients who will someday be in your position. When impartial sponsors conduct clinical trials, there is no reason to hesitate. The upside is large, and the downsides are minimal and carefully monitored. Ask your doctor whether he knows of any such trials that are for people like you.

::

Reversal is common in medicine. You are sure to be offered therapies that are, at the very least, potentially ineffective. Thoughtful questions, asked in the right way, to a doctor who is willing (or can be encouraged) to work with you will expose the riskiest therapies. These questions will also help you to receive proven therapies when they are available and allow you to make informed decisions when they are not.

18

BEYOND DOGMA

:: WHEN RANDOMIZED TRIALS
   ARE UNNECESSARY

OVER THE PRECEDING 17 CHAPTERS, we have tried to make the case that reversal is one of the most important problems in medicine today—if not the most important. The solution to the problem of reversal is to improve the evidence on which medical practice is based. The reversal of widely accepted medical practices can be costly, challenging, contentious, and even injurious. Anyone who has followed the medical news and come away confused should feel vindicated. Medical news is confusing because medical practitioners are confused about the weight of evidence that should be present before adopting a therapy. In our research, we found that that just over half (56 percent) of authors of observational studies in top-tier medical journals believed their data should change medical practice. However, as we have demonstrated over the course of this book, observational studies are unreliable, and trusting them has led to notorious missteps in medicine.

In chapters 14 to 16, we presented our best ideas on how to solve the problem. Currently, doing randomized trials is difficult, costly, and complicated—facts compounded by the indifference of most patients toward participating in these trials. Our solution calls for randomized controlled trials to test every treatment decision we make. Day-to-day medical care should not just have randomized trials as a garnish—that sprig of parsley next to your steak—but should have randomized trials embedded throughout. To accomplish this, we have to create a culture in which demonstrating that a treatment works is an absolute necessity prior to approval and widespread adoption. The default process should be that consenting patients are enrolled in randomized trials, designed by impartial sponsors. By combining a burden-of-proof philosophy with the nudge principle, we could achieve the right model: a medical system in which every patient is treated with practices that we know work and every untested practice is tested in a randomized trial. This is our vision for medicine.

Fundamentalism in all forms, however, is bad. We recognize that in the near term at least (and in some situations for far longer), practices not supported by randomized controlled trials must exist. As clinicians, we are aware that there needs to be wiggle room—we will need to continue to make some decisions without a solid evidence base. However, we hope that this necessity, one that is now the norm, will be restricted to a few situations, such as when a patient with a rare condition is critically ill, when a patient has a truly unique problem, and during diagnostic evaluations.

SITUATIONS THAT ARE BOTH DIRE AND RARE

Every physician occasionally cares for a patient whose condition is truly dire. Depending on where the doctor practices, these situations might be rare or painfully common. Consider one of the common ones. Pulmonary embolism, which we discussed in chapter 16, occurs when a blood clot, typically from the legs, has traveled to the lungs. Usually this problem is accompanied by chest pain and shortness of breath and is treated relatively easily. However, if the clot is massive in size, a pulmonary embolism can strain the heart as it struggles to pump blood past the clot, and cardiac arrest can result. This situation is dire with odds of death higher than anyone would be willing to bear. This is an uncommon occurrence but, in a large hospital, not a rare one. Several strategies have been implemented to treat these patients. Some doctors will send a patient to have open-heart surgery in an attempt to remove the clot. Others will deliver a powerful clot-busting drug via an intravenous infusion. Still other doctors will choose to deliver the same drug, but by threading a catheter right up against the clot—with the hopes of avoiding the catastrophic bleeding that can result from the clot-buster. Most commonly, doctors simply provide basic anticoagulation, the usual treatment for emboli that are not imminently dangerous, allowing the body's own clot-busting systems to do the bulk of the work.

The last choice here—anticoagulation alone—is the best-supported strategy. The other interventions might work, but they are not yet supported by robust randomized trials, and each of them carries real risks. For these situations—dire but not particularly rare—the model we outlined in previous chapters is best. We should do only what we know is beneficial, and each of the more experimental strategies should be tested in randomized trials (using the burden of proof as a guide and the nudge principle to optimize enrollment).

Too often, however, situations are both dire and rare. A patient with an unusual cancer, who is receiving a novel therapy, develops fevers and begins to decline. He becomes delirious. Despite the doctors' best efforts, including broad-spectrum antibiotics and antifungals to treat infections that might be causing the fevers, the patient does not improve and the cause of his decline (and the appropriate solution) remains a mystery. A consulting doctor suggests further suppressing the patient's already compromised immune system. Maybe this makes sense: the fevers could be a response to the novel therapy. Maybe this course is dangerous: if there is an infection, further weakening the immune system might prove deadly. There are no clinical trials to guide us. Do the doctors give it a shot?

In these cases, when a patient's condition is deteriorating, and when the cause is neither clear nor typical, it is reasonable to suspend the burden-of-proof principle and do what seems reasonable. Recently, a team in Philadelphia genetically engineered an immune cell to attack cancer. Patients developed unrelenting fevers and illness after the infusion of these cells. On a hunch, they tried powerful immune blockers. In these cases, the patients got better. Did the drugs help? Possibly, yes. At a minimum, no one could fault the doctors for trying something unproven in this situation.

The tricky part about dire and rare situations is that dire and rare are both relative terms. Dying of cancer is often dire, but for the most part, doctors should not just try random drugs hoping for a cure. In fact, one of the charges of the U.S. FDA is to prevent dying people from taking a remedy that is not very likely to help them and far more likely to hurt them. Dying can often lead to desperation, and desperate people need doctors to counsel them against futile and foolish actions. At the same time, there is a part of human nature that says you have to try something for a patient who is young (another relative term) and is dying of something you do not quite understand. Physicians need to be free and willing to improvise in situations that are dire and rare. However, if that dire situation begins to become a more common one, researchers and clinicians must design a trial to test the interventions.

The frequency of medical reversal should inspire us toward a medical system that reliably improves human health. At the same time, in certain circumstances doctors need to be free to improvise. It is difficult to watch someone suffer or die and it is all the more difficult when that death is untimely or inexplicable. In such cases, the burden of proof should be a bit flexible. However, doctors should try to find commonalities among the dire conditions and use clinical trials to discover successful interventions. Someday, the team in Philadelphia may come to realize that their predicament is not as uncommon as it once was. It may come to be more like the case of massive pulmonary emboli. When that time comes, we should start thinking about how to test what succeeded in a pinch to make sure that it is truly beneficial.

UNIQUE CASES

One of the greatest accomplishments in medicine has been our ability to recognize patterns. For thousands of years, doctors have noticed commonalities among the people they treat and, in the process, identified several thousand diagnoses. With each year, we improve upon this—finding parsimonious genetic or physiological causes of complex diseases. In 1981, for instance, just five men with an unusual pneumonia led doctors to suspect that a new illness was emerging. That illness, of course, was AIDS.

And yet, despite our remarkable ability to find patterns, the complexity that is the human body in health and disease has prevented us from figuring it all out. There are certainly diseases that have yet to be named, and some of the diseases that are presently included in our textbooks will turn out to be syndromes—collections of signs and symptoms—rather than the product of precise physiological defects. Sometimes patients have truly unique conditions or, more commonly, unique constellations of problems. A patient may have a neuroendocrine tumor (a rare cancer) and also have acute kidney failure requiring dialysis. A patient with hemophilia, a bleeding disorder, may also develop an aneurysm (a fragile swelling) of an artery in the brain. These are tough cases. Pragmatic randomized trials, those that try to reflect the real-world populations, are important, but even they are unlikely to fully guide us when the situation is unique.

When treating patients whose problems are unique, physicians need to start with what is known. How do we approach an aneurysm in a patient with hemophilia? We start by considering the surgical approach used to treat this condition in people who do not have the bleeding disorder. Then we begin to weigh in the hemophilia. Can that disease be controlled during surgery and in the postoperative period? What is the excess risk of bleeding in patients with hemophilia? We must include those issues into the risk-benefit calculations.

This is the sort of thinking that doctors are good at. However, when we say "good at," we mean good at thinking that way, not necessarily good at getting the conclusions right. It is impossible to know whether doctors get these difficult cases right (even on average). We can all point to a case for which the result was favorable and in which we are proud of our decision making, but we cannot really say that it was our decision making that led to the good outcome. We can imagine creative ways to test, generally, how best to take care of patients with unique cases. For example: is it better to have the decisions made by a specialist in that disorder, or a specialist in evidence-based medicine, or a doctor with training in risk assessment? (Remember the superspecialists of chapter 14.) A randomized trial of many patients with unique problems could answer these questions but will not provide direction on how to care for an individual in a unique situation. In these cases, doctors will always need to make decisions in an unsystematic way.

Thus, taking care of patients with unique issues is another area in which it is acceptable to suspend the burden of proof. In the years to come, randomized controlled trials will allow us to apply evidence to patients with a broader array of medical problems, but there will always be patients in unique situations, for whom doctors will need to make educated guesses.

DIAGNOSTIC TESTING

Throughout this book, most of the examples of reversal we discussed had to do with treating a patient. A person has a diagnosed ailment and her doctor must decide among treatment options. Some of these options might not be supported by evidence, and if one of these interventions is eventually found wanting, then we will have an example of reversal. Much of clinical medicine, however, happens before the point where treatment is prescribed. The diagnostic process occurs when a person is taken from a complaint to a diagnosis. It is an aspect of medicine that could be far more evidence-based, but this process sometimes also needs to exist outside the strictest demands of the burden of proof.

When a patient comes into the hospital with severe abdominal pain, doctors use clinical reasoning to make a diagnosis. They develop hypotheses based on who the patient is (a 20-year-old man or a 75-year-old woman) and then test these hypotheses. The tests begin with history questions—Where exactly is the pain? Have you had this pain before? Physical examination maneuvers come next: inspection, auscultation, palpation, and percussion—the four pillars of examination. And then laboratory, radiological, or even more invasive tests are done. At each stage, the doctor considers the likelihood of a diagnosis and then revises that likelihood based on the test results. When diagnoses are easy, it is because the tests (history, physical, laboratory, and so on) are highly predictive. If the overweight, 40-year-old woman with pain in the right upper quadrant of her abdomen tells you, "I always get this pain after I eat a fatty meal," you know she has gallstones.

Much of this process is, in fact, evidence-based. There are data that describe how likely women around this age are to have gallstones. We call this the "pretest probability." There are also data about the test characteristics that describe the accuracy of these diagnostic studies. Knowing these characteristics—the sensitivity (how likely a test is to be positive in people with disease) and the specificity (how likely a test is to be negative in people without disease)—allows doctors to calculate, usually more qualitatively than quantitatively, a "post-test probability," the likelihood of a diagnosis.

You are probably already beginning to realize why the ability to be evidence-based in the diagnostic process is challenging. There may be reasons that the pretest probability that you look up in a book does not apply to your patient. Then there are the test characteristics. Are the test characteristics of your physical examination of the patient's abdomen the same as those reported in a journal article? Probably not. The patient and the doctor are different.

Then there are the tests we do that are more exploratory than diagnostic. If our patient is not a textbook case (such as our overweight, 40-year-old woman with right-upper-quadrant abdominal pain) but a more enigmatic one (a 29-year-old man with nonspecific belly pain), how should the case be approached? After a medical history and physical examination, most doctors start with a battery of blood work: blood counts, blood chemistries, liver-function tests. This strategy is not evidence-based. No one has tested in a randomized fashion whether obtaining blood counts or chemistries improves the outcomes of patients with abdominal pain. However, we do it because it is often a helpful part of the process. It gives the doctor a very general idea of a person's health. It might alter the pretest probability of a disease the doctor considered highly improbable. It might provide practical information—knowing the kidney function will be useful in deciding on the next test.

Another issue with trying to study diagnostic tests is that the end points are not as clear as those that exist in studies of therapy. A new treatment for back pain should be evaluated to see whether it helps back pain, but what should the end point be for a new diagnostic test for back pain? The most dogmatic advocate of evidence-based medicine would say that the test is beneficial only if it improves back pain. But common sense tells us that we use diagnostic tests for many reasons. A test might be done to choose later tests, to reassure patients, to offer prognostic information, to evaluate the effectiveness of therapy. These are very difficult end points to study.

All that said, diagnostic medicine should not be an evidence-free zone. There are tests being done that seem to have no role in a well-considered diagnostic process. When such tests are performed routinely, you do not know whether it is because the doctor is practicing defensive medicine, not thinking carefully, or just trying to pad his paycheck. Ultrasound images of the carotid arteries (two of the three arteries supplying the brain) are routinely done in many hospitals as part of the evaluation of patients who have fainted. There is no reason to routinely do this test, and randomized controlled trials could prove that this test is unnecessary in the vast majority of patients. Trials should be done for diagnostic strategies such as this, tests that are routinely employed but whose efficacy is unproved and doubtful. Examination of these practices could have an enormous effect on quality of care and health-care expenditures. When a middle-aged person comes to the emergency room with chest pain that has resolved, hospitals around

America routinely follow the same protocol to detect a heart attack: perform an EKG, a chest X-ray, and blood work. If those tests are negative, most hospitals will pursue some sort of stress test. We should study whether this last test is necessary. Does doing a stress test decrease the rate of missed heart attacks, or does it just run up costs and harm patients by leading to unnecessary, invasive procedures?

There have been some great successes over the past couple of decades in proving the best way to evaluate some very common complaints. Studies have tested how to approach patients with complaints as diverse as low-back pain, ankle sprains, and disabling headaches. The studies have yielded "clinical decision rules" that define which patients require evaluation (and what evaluation is necessary) and which patients can be safely observed. The impact of these studies has been enormously beneficial to patients and the health-care system. We can foresee other studies that would allow us to say things like: for any patient over age 75 who comes in with unintentional weight loss, four tests have been shown to improve survival, six tests contribute to the diagnostic workup only 1 percent of the time, and three other tests add nothing other than increased costs.

It is said that diagnosis is more an art than a science. A patient's symptoms can be idiosyncratic—there may be a finite number of diseases, but there are an infinite number of ways that patients manifest these diseases. Doctors reason through cases in diverse ways. Recognizing that this is the case, and understanding that the goals of diagnostic testing are varied, we understand that clinical diagnosis cannot be completely ruled by the outcomes of clinical trials. That said, not all diagnostic practices are acceptable, and patient care will improve if common diagnostic evaluations with clear end points are standardized. Diagnosis is the part of the job that can still lead us into heated arguments with fellow doctors. We recognize that there needs to be room to accommodate this diversity of thinking.

OPTIMIZING MEDICAL CARE

Francis Peabody is one of the most quoted physicians in American medicine. Probably his most repeated line is, "The secret in caring for the patient is to care for the patient." In order to provide good medical care, you have to have the patient's best interests at heart. By and large, doctors have their hearts in the right place. We all want to do what is right for the people who walk through our doors. Yet, we tend to believe that our biological understanding of disease translates into choosing therapies that work. But as we have seen repeatedly in this book, not biological understanding, not common sense, not observational studies, and not even small, single-center randomized controlled trials are sufficient to conclude that a medical practice works. Although our hearts are in the right place, our heads do not always get it right.

We must also confront the uncomfortable fact that in medicine today, financial incentives bias us. Doctors come to believe—maybe they fool themselves into believing—that a procedure or test that is logical and happens to be well-reimbursed also benefits their patients. We want to believe the practice works, and money can corrupt our thinking.

We must also acknowledge that a bias toward adopting practices prematurely is shared by nearly all the players in health care: researchers and innovators, the drug and device industry, and practicing doctors. Professionally or financially, they all profit from new practices. As a result, regulatory agencies are under pressure to approve more products more quickly. We cannot begin to count the number of articles we have read criticizing the FDA for its excessive caution. As we have tried to convince you, there are good reasons for regulators to be cautious and set a high standard for approval.

Finally, we must recognize that the amount of funding available to study the effectiveness of medical practices is much smaller than the amount of funding available to pay for the untested medical practices. The entire budget of the National Institutes of Health is around $30 billion. Not a small sum, but nothing compared the $550 billion budget of the Centers for Medicare and Medicaid. Our commitment to studying what we do is not nearly where it should be.

For these reasons, our medical system is too tolerant of unproven practices. Doctors are too comfortable recommending a practice without real knowledge of whether it is helping or hurting patients. People are too willing to accept practices that seem like they should help. When a medical reversal does occur, most physicians consider it an exception to the rule. However, as we demonstrated in chapter 7, it may be that nearly half of physicians' treatments are untested practices and simply do not work. Medical reversals are everywhere.

We need a culture change in medicine. We need to recommit to evidence-based medicine and realize that it is the only rational way to provide care. In this book we have provided a few suggestions for ways we can improve. We do not advocate that these recommendations be immediately implemented but that they be carefully considered, alongside recommendations proposed by other thoughtful analysts, and tested in prospective trials. As we move forward, we must recognize that drastic and dramatic change can often be harmful. We acknowledge that there will be areas of medicine in which, for now, we must tolerate the status quo. As we go through the house of medicine and clean up each room, we have to prioritize. This chapter is our best guess regarding which rooms should be cleaned last.

Now is the time to begin cleaning.

ACKNOWLEDGMENTS

VKP AND ASC

Two authors were nowhere nearly enough to bring this book to completion. Many smart, talented, and hardworking people have collaborated with us in our work on medical reversal. These collaborators included Andrae Vandross, Jason Rho, Victor Gall, Joel Jorgenson, Senthil Selvaraj, Nancy Ho, Caitlin Toomey, Jacob Chacko, Steven Quinn, Durga Borkar, and Michael Cheung. We are especially indebted to Rita Redberg, who, in her position as editor of *JAMA Internal Medicine,* supported us from our earliest investigations and has been a tireless advocate of evidence-based practice. John P. A. Ioannidis, a pioneer in the study of medical research, has been a generous collaborator.

Alex Lickerman, Eric Oliver, and Thea Goodman helped guide us when we first began work on this book. Stephany Evans, at FinePrint Literary Management, recognized the potential of this project and worked tirelessly on our behalf. At Johns Hopkins University Press, thank you to the reviewers who so carefully read and commented on the manuscript. Jackie Wehmueller encouraged and supported us in this project and helped us arrive at a title.

VKP

I am grateful to the people who taught me to think critically about the world around us, and those who showed me how beautiful medicine can be, particularly Marcia Aldrich, Sanjeeve Balasubramaniam, Jean Burns, Fred Gifford, Robert Hirschtick, David Horn, Barnett Kramer, Peter Mayock, H. G. Munshi, David Neely, James Nelson, John Sherrick, Scott Stern, Scot Yoder, and many others whom I am forgetting. I also thank my friends, who constantly challenged my thinking: Andrae Vandross, David Straus, William Thistlethwaite, Tim Howes, and Nathan Lord. My deep gratitude to Dr. Antonio Tito Fojo, senior investigator and program director at the National Cancer Institute. Tito Fojo taught me to be a better researcher, a better critic, and a better oncologist. He invested so much in me, and has bailed me out of jail more times than I deserved. Adam Cifu has been the perfect partner in crime over these years, all of the above, and a dear friend. Finally, the people who have been with me through everything: my parents, Padma and Ram, who deserve credit for everything good within me and still teach me what it means to be wise and compassionate; my brother Karthik, whose kindness and cleverness amaze me; and my wife, Nancy, who brings out the best in me.

ASC

I am indebted to the colleagues and mentors who inspired and encouraged both my love of medicine and my interest in the evidence on which we base our practice. During my training, Carol Bates, Booker Bush, and physicians in the Division of General Internal Medicine at the Beth Israel Hospital in Boston taught me what it means to be a specialist in general medicine and how to critically analyze clinical research. Their wisdom and enthusiasm have been with me ever since. At the University of Chicago, Halina Brukner has guided me through the world of academic medicine from the start. Diane Altkorn and Scott Stern have been both colleagues and mentors for the past 18 years. For me, our work together laid the foundation of this book. The Pritzker students have always been refreshingly challenging in their intellectual curiosity and energy. Final thanks to Anne Cifu, who provided me a few of the writers' genes from the Craig family; Vinayak Prasad, who is the perfect collaborator—generous, energetic, creative, and thick-skinned; and Sarah Stein, who has been everything—from most ardent supporter to most critical (in every sense) editor.

APPENDIX

THIS APPENDIX SUMMARIZES studies appearing in the *New England Journal of Medicine* between 2001 and 2010 that contradicted accepted practices. These are not occasions when a newer, better therapy was announced, and they are not negative studies of potential innovations; they are reversals—each study provided evidence that overturned a practice that was already in use, suggesting that what had come before that practice was better.

Most of the studies are unambiguous examples of reversal. Studies 31, 37, and 38 overturned the practice of prescribing estrogen-replacement therapy. Study 85 is the COURAGE trial that argued against placing stents in people with stable coronary-artery disease. Studies 124 and 125 proved that vertebroplasty was ineffective. Some are examples of less complete reversals, where it is proved that an existing practice or therapy is much less effective than believed. Numbers 40 and 136 are in this category. Other studies looked at two therapies that were considered equivalent and established that one was superior (studies 52 and 133).

Among the studies listed below are novel types of reversal that we recognized. Sometimes an effective therapy has been withheld because of unsupported concerns about its safety. Studies 1, 2, and 68 are examples of research proving that such concerns were spurious and allowing an effective therapy to be used once again. A few of the reversals can be attributed to the evolution of medicine. In study 48, for example, a therapy that had been proved effective is later shown to be ineffective. This reversal probably occurred not because the initial data were flawed but because, in the intervening years, new therapies were developed that overwhelmed the small benefit of the initial intervention. Some of the studies overturn new practices (for example, study 60), while others overturn practices that had been used for a half century (studies 51, 141, and 142). On the whole, the list suggests that a great many medical practices—practices sometimes supported by professional guidelines and paid for by major insurance providers—are later shown not to work.

For those who are interested, greater detail about each study is provided in the supplemental material of our original article, "A Decade of Reversal" (see the list of references for the chapter 7 section). The supplemental material is available at www.mayoclinicproceedings.org/cms/attachment/2007391767/2029532464/mmc2.pdf.

	STUDY	DATE OF PUBLICATION	SUMMARY
1	Vaccinations and the risk of relapse in multiple sclerosis	2/1/01	Long-standing concerns about vaccinations preceding the onset or relapse of multiple sclerosis led to clinicians' reluctance to give vaccinations to these patients. This study proved no increased risk of relapse in the two-month period immediately following tetanus, hepatitis B, or influenza vaccination.
2	Hepatitis B vaccination and the risk of multiple sclerosis	2/1/01	On a topic related to the previous study, this study disproved the relationship between vaccination and the development of multiple sclerosis.
3	Lack of effect of induction of hypothermia after acute brain injury	2/22/01	This study found that the practice of cooling patients after brain injury, which had been done for decades, is not beneficial.
4	Initial plasma HIV-1 RNA levels and progression to AIDS in women and men	3/8/01	This study contradicted a common decision-making practice concerning when to start medications for HIV in women.

STUDY	DATE OF PUBLICATION	SUMMARY
5 The teratogenicity of anticonvulsant drugs	4/12/01	Two medical textbooks and one review article have doubted that anticonvulsants taken during pregnancy are more teratogenic than epilepsy itself. This large study found the opposite: anticonvulsants during pregnancy increase the risk of fetal malformation.
6 Effect of early or delayed insertion of tympanostomy tubes for persistent otitis media on developmental outcomes at the age of three years	4/19/01	Guidelines recommended insertion of ear tubes in a child with an ear infection of greater than three months' duration because of concerns that associated conductive hearing loss might lead to poor developmental outcomes. This study did not find any benefit in early tube placement.
7 The effect of chelation therapy with succimer on neuropsychological development in children exposed to lead	5/10/01	This study looked at an accepted therapy for children with moderately elevated blood lead levels and found no benefit.
8 Long-term effects of indomethacin prophylaxis in extremely-low-birth-weight infants	6/28/01	This study showed that a preventive therapy, commonly used in infants with extremely low birth weights, did not improve survival without neurosensory impairment at 18 months.
9 Two controlled trials of antibiotic treatment in patients with persistent symptoms and a history of Lyme disease	7/12/01	These studies showed no benefit of a controversial but often-utilized treatment: a prolonged course of antibiotics for patients with persistent symptoms of Lyme disease.
10 Three months versus one year of oral anticoagulant therapy for idiopathic deep venous thrombosis	7/19/01	When treating blood clots in the legs, longer therapy is often considered better. This trial showed that a prolonged course of therapy delayed but did not reduce the risk for a recurrent clot.

STUDY	DATE OF PUBLICATION	SUMMARY
11 Failure of metronida-zole to prevent preterm delivery among pregnant women with asymptomatic Trichomonas vaginalis infection	8/16/01	Pregnant women are often screened for an asymptomatic vag-inal infection (which is treated if found), in the hopes of decreasing the risk of preterm birth. This trial showed that this practice actually increases the risk of preterm birth.
12 Effect of prone position-ing on the survival of patients with acute respi-ratory failure	8/23/01	This study overturned a practice of positioning ICU patients prone while they are on a ventilator.
13 Medical treatment for neurocysticercosis characterized by giant subarachnoid cysts	9/20/01	This trial showed that surgical therapy for a parasitic brain infec-tion may not be as widely neces-sary as was the accepted practice.
14 Naltrexone in the treat-ment of alcohol depen-dence	12/13/01	In this multicenter, double-blind, placebo-controlled study, a com-monly used therapy for alcohol dependence was shown to be ineffective.
15 Comparison of two diets for the prevention of recurrent stones in idio-pathic hypercalciuria	1/10/02	This trial showed that a low-calcium diet, commonly recom-mended for kidney stones, actually increased the risk of stones.
16 Frequency of uterine contractions and the risk of spontaneous preterm delivery	1/24/02	This study added to evidence that monitoring for frequent contrac-tions (commonly done on labor and delivery wards) is not helpful in decreasing the rate of preterm delivery.
17 Screening of infants and mortality due to neuro-blastoma	4/04/02	Studies 17 and 18 overturned a screening test, adopted in Japan, for a childhood cancer.
18 Neuroblastoma screening at one year of age	4/04/02	See study 17.
19 Immediate repair com-pared with surveillance of small abdominal aortic aneurysms	5/09/02	This trial raised doubts about a common threshold for when ab-dominal aortic aneurysms should be repaired.

	STUDY	DATE OF PUBLICATION	SUMMARY
20	Intranasal mupirocin to prevent postoperative Staphylococcus aureus infections	6/13/02	This randomized controlled trial overturned a common practice of eradicating nasal colonization with Staphylococcus aureus before surgery.
21	A controlled trial of arthroscopic surgery for osteoarthritis of the knee	7/11/02	As discussed in chapter 3, this study found that arthroscopic surgery for osteoarthritis of the knee is ineffective.
22	Twenty-five-year follow-up of a randomized trial comparing radical mastectomy, total mastectomy, and total mastectomy followed by irradiation	8/22/02	In a follow-up of an older reversal, this trial failed to show benefit for a more aggressive surgery, which dominated medicine in the 20th century.
23	Sex-based differences in the effect of digoxin for the treatment of heart failure	10/31/02	Contradicting recommendations by the American College of Cardiology, the European Society of Cardiology, and the Heart Failure Society of America, this analysis found that digitalis increases the rate of death among women.
24	Antimicrobial treatment in diabetic women with asymptomatic bacteriuria	11/14/02	Some groups recommended screening and treating women with diabetes for the asymptomatic presence of bacteria in urine specimens. This randomized trial found that this practice does not reduce complications or delay the onset of symptomatic infection.
25	A comparison of rate control and rhythm control in patients with atrial fibrillation	12/5/02	Studies 25 and 26 were landmark studies showing that a lesser intervention for atrial fibrillation, a common arrhythmia, was as effective as a more aggressive approach.
26	A comparison of rate control and rhythm control in patients with recurrent persistent atrial fibrillation	12/5/02	See study 25.

	STUDY	DATE OF PUBLICATION	SUMMARY
27	A randomized, controlled trial of the use of pulmonary-artery catheters in high-risk surgical patients	1/2/03	This trial added to data questioning the use of a common monitoring device, the pulmonary artery catheter, in elderly, high-risk patients.
28	Imaging studies after a first febrile urinary tract infection in young children	1/16/03	This study suggested that at least part of our evaluation of young children with urinary tract infections is unnecessary.
29	Serum retinol levels and the risk of fracture	1/23/03	This suggests that some nations' practice of vitamin A supplementation and food fortification ought to be reevaluated, since high levels of vitamin A are associated with fractures.
30	Factors associated with progression of carcinoid heart disease	3/13/03	This trial showed that an intervention for a rare tumor was associated with significant harm.
31	Effects of estrogen plus progestin on health-related quality of life	5/8/03	On the topic that is probably the best-known example of reversal, this Women's Health Initiative study found that the use of estrogen plus progestin did not improve women's quality of life. There was no significant effect on health, vitality, mental health, depressive symptoms, or sexual satisfaction in women receiving the hormones as compared to placebo. This study is discussed in chapter 9.
32	Involved-field radiotherapy for advanced Hodgkin's lymphoma	6/12/03	This study suggested an important change in the treatment of advanced Hodgkin's lymphoma.
33	Conventional adjuvant chemotherapy with or without high-dose chemotherapy and autologous stem-cell transplantation in high-risk breast cancer	7/3/03	In a rapidly changing field, this study showed that a commonly used, more aggressive intervention reduced risk of relapse of breast cancer but did not improve mortality.

	STUDY	DATE OF PUBLICATION	SUMMARY
34	A multicenter, random-ized, double-blind, con-trolled trial of nebulized epinephrine in infants with acute bronchiolitis	7/3/03	This trial compared nebulized epinephrine with placebo in 194 infants with bronchiolitis and showed that there was no significant difference in length of hospitalization, a more meaning-ful end point than those used in previous trials that supported this therapy.
35	Evaluation of imperme-able covers for bedding in patients with allergic rhinitis	7/17/03	The encasement of bedding with impermeable covers has been recommended for the treatment of allergic rhinitis. Although this study showed that this interven-tion reduced allergen emission from mattresses, it had no effect on clinical outcomes.
36	Control of exposure to mite allergen and allergen-impermeable bed covers for adults with asthma	7/17/03	Similar to study 35, this double-blind, randomized, placebo-controlled trial of more than 1,100 patients found no benefit on any clinical or physiological outcome for this practice.
37	Estrogen plus progestin and the risk of coronary heart disease	8/7/03	Following study 31, studies 37 and 38 furthered the evidence that estrogen-replacement therapy is ineffective.
38	Hormone therapy and the progression of coronary-artery atherosclerosis in postmenopausal women	8/7/03	See study 37.
39	Outcomes at school age after postnatal dexameth-asone therapy for lung disease of prematurity	3/25/04	This study raised serious concerns about one of the standard thera-pies for premature newborns.

STUDY	DATE OF PUBLICATION	SUMMARY
40 C-reactive protein and other circulating markers of inflammation in the prediction of coronary heart disease	4/1/04	Measuring C-reactive protein (CRP) to evaluate for the risk of coronary atherosclerosis had been supported by numerous guidelines. This study showed that CRP was only a moderate predictor of the risk of coronary-artery disease and added only marginally to the predictive value of established risk factors. The authors called for guidelines to be reviewed on the basis of their findings.
41 The influence of resection and aneuploidy on mortality in oral leukoplakia	4/1/04	This article suggested a reversal in the treatment of a precancerous lesion, but the article was retracted when suspicions arose that the data contained in the paper were falsified.
42 A comparison of high-dose and standard-dose epinephrine in children with cardiac arrest	4/22/04	This study overturned recommendations from the American Heart Association for pediatric advanced life support.
43 Open mesh versus laparoscopic mesh repair of inguinal hernia	4/29/04	This study argued that the older, open method for repairing hernias is superior to the newer, laparoscopic approach.
44 Folate therapy and in-stent restenosis after coronary stenting	6/24/04	This study suggested that folate therapy (actually folic acid, vitamin B_6, and vitamin B_{12}) is ineffective in preventing the failure of stenting procedures for coronary-artery disease.
45 Methylprednisolone, valacyclovir, or the combination for vestibular neuritis	7/22/04	It was common practice to prescribe an antiviral medication and steroid for vestibular neuritis until this study showed that only the steroid, and not the antiviral medication, improved recovery.

	STUDY	DATE OF PUBLICATION	SUMMARY
46	Lumpectomy plus tamoxifen with or without irradiation in women 70 years of age or older with early breast cancer	9/2/04	This study suggested that withholding radiation therapy for a group of older women with breast cancer does not worsen their outcomes.
47	Fresh whole blood versus reconstituted blood for pump priming in heart surgery in infants	10/14/04	This study suggested that a novel and physiologically sensible transfusion strategy was not better than the former standard in infants undergoing cardio-pulmonary bypass surgery.
48	Angiotensin converting–enzyme inhibition in stable coronary-artery disease	11/11/04	This is a controversial reversal in which a former standard (use of ACE-inhibitor medications in patients with vascular disease) was overturned. The failure of these medications to work in this study might be less a reversal and more the result of improvements in the care of these patients.
49	Secondary surgical cytoreduction for advanced ovarian carcinoma	12/9/04	This study strongly suggested that less aggressive surgical care in a subset of patients with ovarian cancer is as effective as recently adopted, more aggressive care.
50	Coronary-artery revascularization before elective major vascular surgery	12/30/04	This randomized, multicenter VA trial revealed that a common intervention, coronary-artery revascularization in patients with stable disease who are scheduled to undergo elective vascular surgery, did not offer any benefit.

	STUDY	DATE OF PUBLICATION	SUMMARY
51	Mild intraoperative hypothermia during surgery for intracranial aneurysm	1/13/05	Hypothermia was found to be helpful as a neurosurgical adjunct in 1955. At the time of this publication, the technique was being used in nearly 50 percent of aneurysm surgeries. This large randomized study showed no improvement in neurological outcomes with hypothermia and an increase in bacterial infections.
52	Clopidogrel versus aspirin and esomeprazole to prevent recurrent ulcer bleeding	1/20/05	For patients who have had gastrointestinal bleeding while on aspirin, guidelines recommended either the use of clopidogrel or the addition of a proton pump inhibitor to aspirin as equivalent strategies. This study showed that aspirin plus the proton pump inhibitor esomeprazole was far superior to clopidogrel in preventing future ulcer bleeding.
53	The risk of cesarean delivery with neuraxial analgesia given early versus late in labor	2/17/05	The American College of Obstetrics and Gynecology recommended that epidural anesthesia be delayed until cervical dilation had reached at least 4 centimeters. This study showed that early and late epidural anesthesia are equivalent strategies.
54	UK controlled trial of intrapleural streptokinase for pleural infection	3/3/05	Although guidelines suggested that intrapleural fibrinolytics helped the drainage of infected pleural effusions (fluid collections around the lungs) and reduced the need for surgical drainage, this study found no benefit in the important end points.

	STUDY	DATE OF PUBLICATION	SUMMARY
55	Cardiovascular events associated with rofecoxib in a colorectal adenoma chemoprevention trial	3/17/05	This study, and studies 56 and 57, have been widely reported on. All three suggest that selective COX-2 inhibitors, widely prescribed pain medications that include Celebrex and Vioxx, might increase the risk of cardiovascular events.
56	Cardiovascular risk associated with celecoxib in a clinical trial for colorectal adenoma prevention	3/17/05	See study 55.
57	Complications of the COX-2 inhibitors parecoxib and valdecoxib after cardiac surgery	3/17/05	See study 55.
58	Comparison of warfarin and aspirin for symptomatic intracranial arterial stenosis	3/31/05	Some doctors use the anticoagulant warfarin in the treatment of intracranial arterial stenosis. This study showed that warfarin therapy was associated with higher rates of adverse events and no benefit compared to aspirin.
59	Long-term outcomes of coronary-artery bypass grafting versus stent implantation	5/26/05	Patients with narrowing of multiple coronary arteries have traditionally been treated with coronary-artery bypass surgery. Recently, percutaneous coronary intervention (PCI, or stenting) has been increasingly used to treat these patients. This observational study found that bypass surgery is still superior to PCI.
60	Hydroxyurea compared with anagrelide in high-risk essential thrombocythemia	7/7/05	Anagrelide was a new drug that was gaining use for patients with essential thrombocythemia—abnormally high blood platelets. This trial showed that the traditional therapy, hydroxyurea plus aspirin, is superior.

	STUDY	DATE OF PUBLICATION	SUMMARY
61	Inhaled nitric oxide for premature infants with severe respiratory failure	7/7/05	This large, multicenter, randomized trial showed that the use of inhaled nitric oxide was ineffective in infants weighing less than 1,500 grams at birth. This treatment was previously supported by a single-center study.
62	An evaluation of echinacea angustifolia in experimental rhinovirus infections	7/28/05	As discussed in chapter 6, this study showed that echinacea provides no benefit in symptom duration or severity with rhinovirus infection (the common cold).
63	Developmental outcomes after early or delayed insertion of tympanostomy tubes	8/11/05	Similar to study 6, this study showed no difference in development between prompt and delayed placement of ear tubes.
64	Amnioinfusion for the prevention of the meconium aspiration syndrome	9/1/05	This trial contradicted a meta-analysis by finding that infusion of saline into the amniotic cavity of high-risk pregnant women had no benefit for preventing meconium aspiration syndrome (or other major maternal or neonatal disorders).
65	Early invasive versus selectively invasive management for acute coronary syndromes	9/15/05	In a rapidly changing field, this study suggested that a common, more invasive strategy for patients with unstable coronary disease might not be superior.
66	Long-term vasodilator therapy in patients with severe aortic regurgitation	9/29/05	Although guidelines suggested the use of the drug nifedipine for asymptomatic patients with severe aortic regurgitation (a heart-valve disease), this study found no benefit of the treatment in reducing or delaying the need for valve-replacement surgery.

	STUDY	DATE OF PUBLICATION	SUMMARY
67	Continuous positive airway pressure for central sleep apnea and heart failure	11/10/05	This study was a controversial reversal, in that although the study showed numerous benefits for the use of continuous positive airway pressure (CPAP) for treating central sleep apnea in patients with heart failure, it showed neither a mortality benefit nor a quality-of-life benefit.
68	A trial of contraceptive methods in women with systemic lupus erythematosus	12/15/05	Oral contraceptives are often withheld from patients with lupus for fear that they might worsen the disease. Studies 68 and 69 showed that the use of oral contraceptives does not increase the incidence of lupus flares.
69	Combined oral contraceptives in women with systemic lupus erythematosus	12/15/05	See study 68.
70	The risk associated with aprotinin in cardiac surgery	1/26/06	This trial showed that a drug used for patients having surgery for myocardial infarction was associated with increased risk of renal failure, myocardial infarction or heart failure, and stroke.
71	Clozapine alone versus clozapine and risperidone with refractory schizophrenia	2/2/06	Often patients with schizophrenia are given multiple drugs to control symptoms. This study showed that the combination of two commonly used drugs was no better than one.
72	Saw palmetto for benign prostatic hyperplasia	2/9/06	Although saw palmetto is used by more than 2 million men in the United States for the symptoms of prostate enlargement, this study showed no benefit in multiple outcomes.

	STUDY	DATE OF PUBLICATION	SUMMARY
73	Calcium plus vitamin D supplementation and the risk of fractures	2/16/06	As discussed in chapter 6, this study suggested the commonly used calcium with vitamin D supplementation does not reduce hip fracture and increases the risk of kidney stones.
74	Glucosamine, chondroitin sulfate, and the two in combination for painful knee osteoarthritis	2/23/06	Also discussed in chapter 6, this study showed that glucosamine and chondroitin sulfate, alone or in combination, did not reduce pain in patients with osteoarthritis of the knee.
75	Efficacy and safety of corticosteroids for persistent acute respiratory distress syndrome	4/20/06	This study overturned the practice of using steroids to treat patients with acute respiratory distress syndrome, a common complication of critically ill patients.
76	Pulmonary-artery versus central venous catheter to guide treatment of acute lung injury	5/25/06	Similar to study 27, this study called into question the utility of the pulmonary artery catheter.
77	A controlled trial of homocysteine lowering and cognitive performance	6/29/06	Because observational studies suggested that people with low levels of plasma homocysteine retain better cognitive function, some clinicians have prescribed the vitamins folate, B_{12}, and B_6. This double-blind, placebo-controlled, randomized clinical trial showed that this intervention is not beneficial.
78	Effectiveness of atypical antipsychotic drugs in patients with Alzheimer's disease	10/12/06	This important study demonstrated the high incidence of adverse effects caused by medications commonly used to treat psychosis, aggression, and agitation in patients with Alzheimer's disease.

	STUDY	DATE OF PUBLICATION	SUMMARY
79	DHEA in elderly women and DHEA or testosterone in elderly men	10/19/06	DHEA and testosterone are widely promoted as supplements. In this placebo-controlled, randomized, double-blind study, men were randomized to placebo, testosterone, or DHEA. Women received either DHEA or placebo. Neither DHEA nor low-dose testosterone were shown to have beneficial effects on body composition, physical performance, insulin sensitivity, or quality of life.
80	Correction of anemia with epoetin alfa in chronic kidney disease	11/16/06	Patients with kidney disease often develop an anemia that can be effectively treated with erythropoiesis-stimulating agents. How aggressively this anemia should be treated was unclear, and both guidelines and practice tended toward more aggressive therapy. This trial showed that less aggressive therapy was equally effective.
81	Coronary intervention for persistent occlusion after myocardial infarction	12/7/06	Patients with persistent total occlusion of a coronary artery after treatment for a myocardial infarction were often treated with stenting. This trial showed that this intervention was no better than optimal medical therapy alone (and might actually be associated with a higher likelihood of recurrent myocardial infarctions).
82	Tympanostomy tubes and developmental outcomes at 9 to 11 years of age	1/18/07	Further follow-up from a study showing no benefit of inserting ear tubes in children with middle-ear infections. (See studies 6 and 63.)
83	Long-term outcomes with drug-eluting stents versus bare-metal stents in Sweden	3/8/07	This study reversed the use of a certain type of stent in a subset of patients with narrowed coronary arteries.

STUDY	DATE OF PUBLICATION	SUMMARY
84 Influence of computer-aided detection on performance of screening mammography	4/5/07	This is an unsettled and highly controversial topic. This study suggested that the adoption of computer-aided detection systems to analyze digitized mammograms was actually associated with reduced accuracy of interpretation.
85 Optimal medical therapy with or without PCI for stable coronary disease	4/12/07	The COURAGE trial, reversing the use of stents for stable coronary-artery disease, is discussed throughout this book.
86 Effectiveness of adjunctive antidepressant treatment for bipolar depression	4/26/07	Although the FDA had not approved standard antidepressants for treatment of bipolar depression, many physicians used them in addition to the more accepted medications. This randomized controlled trial showed that the use of a standard antidepressant as an adjunctive treatment was not associated with better outcomes.
87 Randomized comparison of strategies for reducing treatment in mild persistent asthma	5/17/07	This trial showed that one way of reducing asthma therapy, from an inhaled steroid to montelukast, was ineffective.
88 Effect of rosiglitazone on the risk of myocardial infarction and death from cardiovascular causes	6/14/07	The Avandia controversy was well covered in the press (and discussed briefly in chapter 3). Rosiglitazone was introduced in 1999 and was approved in type 2 diabetes mellitus because of its ability to reduce blood glucose and HbA1c (surrogate outcomes). This meta-analysis found that rosiglitazone was associated with a significant increase in the risk of myocardial infarction.

STUDY	DATE OF PUBLICATION	SUMMARY
89 In vitro fertilization with preimplantation genetic screening	7/5/07	Because of the concern that low pregnancy rates in older women undergoing in vitro fertilization (IVF) may be due to the increased prevalence of chromosomal abnormalities, the use of genetic screening had become increasingly common. This trial comparing IVF with and without preimplantation genetic screening found that screening actually reduced rates of ongoing pregnancies and live births.
90 A multicenter, randomized controlled trial of dexamethasone for bronchiolitis	7/26/07	This trial showed that a single dose of an oral steroid administered in the emergency room, although a common practice, did not reduce the rate of hospital admission or improve either the child's respiratory status after four hours or later outcomes, in children with moderate-to-severe bronchiolitis.
91 Saline or albumin for fluid resuscitation in patients with traumatic brain injury	8/30/07	Because there was no consensus on the best choice of fluids for fluid resuscitation in patients with traumatic brain injury, both albumin and saline were used. This study showed that fluid resuscitation with albumin was associated with higher mortality rates.

	STUDY	DATE OF PUBLICATION	SUMMARY
92	High-dose melphalan versus melphalan plus dexamethasone for AL amyloidosis	9/13/07	At the time of this study, high-dose melphalan with autologous hematopoietic stem-cell rescue was commonly used to treat patients with AL amyloidosis, but transplant-related mortality was high. This randomized trial showed that AL amyloidosis treatment with high-dose melphalan plus autologous hematopoietic stem-cell transplant was not superior to the outcome with standard-dose melphalan plus dexamethasone.
93	Outcomes at 2 years of age after repeat doses of antenatal corticosteroids	9/20/07	Studies 93 and 94 both look at the use of steroids in women before the birth of preterm infants. The studies showed that multiple doses of steroids (which had become common), compared to the standard single dose, reduced neonatal morbidity but did not change survival free of major neurosensory disability or body size at 2 years of age.
94	Long-term outcomes after repeat doses of antenatal corticosteroids	9/20/07	See study 93.
95	Early treatment with prednisolone or acyclovir in Bell's palsy	10/18/07	Because Bell's palsy is thought to be caused by a viral infection and is associated with inflammation, both an antiviral and anti-inflammatory steroids were commonly used in its treatment. This randomized, controlled trial showed that while the steroid significantly improved the chances of complete recovery, the antiviral was not beneficial.

STUDY	DATE OF PUBLICATION	SUMMARY
96 Lung transplantation and survival in children with cystic fibrosis	11/22/07	This study looked at the difficult issue of how to treat the sickest children with cystic fibrosis. Lung transplantation is the most aggressive therapy for end-stage lung disease from cystic fibrosis. This large study showed that lung transplantation improved survival in less than 1 percent of patients with cystic fibrosis and suggested that lung transplantation should not be expected to prolong life.
97 Rosuvastatin in older patients with systolic heart failure	11/29/07	This randomized controlled trial showed that a cholesterol-lowering drug did not reduce the rate of death from cardiovascular causes or death from any cause in patients with systolic heart failure. It did reduce the number of cardiovascular hospitalizations, but this was not the trial's primary end point.
98 Dexamethasone in Vietnamese adolescents and adults with bacterial meningitis	12/13/07	Steroids are commonly added to antibiotics in the treatment of bacterial meningitis. This randomized controlled trial showed that a steroid, dexamethasone, did not significantly improve outcomes in Vietnamese adolescents and adults with bacterial meningitis. (There may be some beneficial effect for patients with biologically proven disease, including those who have previously received antibiotic treatment.)
99 Corticosteroids for bacterial meningitis in adults in sub-Saharan Africa	12/13/07	This study considered the same question in an area of high HIV prevalence. The randomized controlled trial took place in Malawi and showed that dexamethasone did not reduce mortality or morbidity.

	STUDY	DATE OF PUBLICATION	SUMMARY
100	Hydrocortisone therapy for patients with septic shock	1/10/08	This study overturned the use of short-term, high-dose steroids to treat septic shock.
101	Intensive insulin therapy and pentastarch resuscitation in severe sepsis	1/10/08	Another study of patients with sepsis, this one questioned the practice of aggressively controlling blood glucose in these patients. In this study, not only was no mortality benefit noted, but the trial was stopped early because of severe hypoglycemic events leading to prolonged ICU stays.
102	Aprotinin during coronary-artery bypass grafting and risk of death	2/21/08	Studies 102 and 103 showed that aprotinin, used in cardiac surgery to reduce blood loss and maintain platelet function, had greater harms than the previous standard.
103	The effect of aprotinin on outcome after coronary-artery bypass grafting	2/21/08	See study 102.
104	Vasopressin versus norepinephrine infusion in patients with septic shock	2/28/08	This is another trial showing that a new intervention, which was being used clinically to treat ICU patients, was no better than the previous standard.
105	Anesthesia awareness and the bispectral index	3/13/08	The bispectral index (BIS) is an important brain-function monitor for anesthesiologists to prevent sensory perception (patient awareness) during surgery. This trial showed that the monitor resulted neither in lower rates of anesthesia awareness nor in lower use of volatile anesthetic gas.
106	Simvastatin with or without ezetimibe in familial hypercholesterolemia	4/3/08	In this trial, the use of the commonly used drug ezetimibe was found to lower cholesterol but not improve a surrogate end point.

	STUDY	DATE OF PUBLICATION	SUMMARY
107	Metformin versus insulin for the treatment of gestational diabetes	5/8/08	This is a reversal in that a beneficial medication was being withheld because of unfounded concerns. The drug metformin was considered beneficial for treatment for gestational diabetes, but its use became controversial because of the question of adverse perinatal effects. When metformin was compared with insulin in this open-labeled random controlled trial, there was no significant increase in perinatal complications.
108	A comparison of aprotinin and lysine analogues in high-risk cardiac surgery	5/29/08	This is a study, similar to studies 70, 102, and 103, on the negative effects of aprotinin.
109	Intensive blood glucose control and vascular outcomes in patients with type 2 diabetes	6/12/08	This trial (ADVANCE) and the next (ACCORD) both demonstrated that very aggressive control of blood sugar in (at least certain) patients with type 2 diabetes—an approach advocated by many doctors—is not beneficial and carries real risks.
110	Effects of intensive glucose lowering in type 2 diabetes	6/12/08	See study 109.
111	Rhythm control versus rate control for atrial fibrillation and heart failure	6/19/08	Similar to studies 25 and 26, this trial showed that converting patients from atrial fibrillation to sinus rhythm was no better than just controlling their heart rate.

STUDY	DATE OF PUBLICATION	SUMMARY
112 Noninvasive ventilation in acute cardiogenic pulmonary edema	7/10/08	In order to avoid the complications of endotracheal intubation (use of a breathing machine), noninvasive ventilation strategies are often used in patients with heart failure. Although this study demonstrated some improvements with this approach, there was no difference in the effect on short-term mortality between standard oxygen therapy and noninvasive ventilation.
113 A randomized trial of arthroscopic surgery for osteoarthritis of the knee	9/11/08	Similar to study 21, this trial failed to show a benefit of arthroscopic surgery for treatment of osteoarthritis of the knee.
114 Prolonged therapy of advanced chronic hepatitis C with low-dose peginterferon	12/4/08	Given more recent advances, this reversal is unimportant, but at the time it showed that not all means of suppressing the hepatitis C virus would lead to clinically important benefits.
115 Oral prednisolone for preschool children with acute virus-induced wheezing	1/22/09	Several sets of national guidelines recommended that oral corticosteroids be given to preschool-aged children who are brought to a hospital with virus-induced wheezing. This large randomized, double-blind, placebo-controlled trial found no benefit in this approach.
116 Quality of life after late invasive therapy for occluded arteries	2/19/09	This study extended the findings of study 81.
117 Intensive versus conventional glucose control in critically ill patients	3/26/09	Similar to trial 101, this study showed that aggressive control of blood sugar in patients in the intensive care unit actually increased the absolute risk of death at 90 days.

	STUDY	DATE OF PUBLICATION	SUMMARY
118	Mortality results from a randomized prostate-cancer screening trial	3/26/09	The mortality benefit of routine prostate-cancer-specific antigen (PSA) screening continues to be debated but has been accepted practice for two decades. This large, randomized trial failed to detect any mortality benefit of routine screening among American men.
119	Rosuvastatin and cardio-vascular events in patients undergoing hemodialysis	4/2/09	Because of their significant cardio-vascular risk, people on dialysis for kidney failure were often pre-scribed cholesterol-lowering statin medicines. This study found no benefit in the combined end point of myocardial infarction, stroke, or death from cardiovascular causes among these patients, despite significant improvements in LDL cholesterol.
120	Efficacy of esomeprazole for treatment of poorly controlled asthma	4/9/09	Because acid reflux is thought to exacerbate asthma, people with poorly controlled asthma are commonly tested for reflux and, if it is diagnosed, treated. This study found that, despite a substantial incidence of reflux, the addition of reflux treatment did not confer benefit.
121	Cognitive function at 3 years of age after fetal exposure to antiepileptic drugs	4/16/09	Multiple guidelines do not distinguish among antiepileptic drugs used during pregnancy with respect to risk to the fetus. This study found that valproic acid, as compared with other commonly used drugs, was associated with poorer cognitive function in the child, at 3 years of age.

	STUDY	DATE OF PUBLICATION	SUMMARY
122	Early versus delayed provisional eptifibatide in acute coronary syndromes	5/21/09	This study looked at a drug recommended before angiography in patients with myocardial infarction and found that this early use was not superior to its traditional use after angiography.
123	Endoscopic versus open vein-graft harvesting in coronary-artery bypass surgery	7/16/09	Endoscopic harvesting of the saphenous vein for use in coronary-artery bypass surgery had become popular because it eliminated the need for the long incisions associated with open harvesting, reduced wound infections, decreased postoperative pain, and shortened the length of stay in the hospital. This study, however, showed that endoscopic harvesting resulted in higher rates of vein-graft failure at 12 to 18 months and, at three years, higher rates of death, myocardial infarction, or repeat revascularization.
124	A randomized trial of vertebroplasty for painful osteoporotic vertebral fractures	8/6/09	Studies 124 and 125 demonstrated the failure of vertebroplasty, discussed extensively in chapter 1.
125	A randomized trial of vertebroplasty for osteoporotic spinal fractures	8/6/09	See study 124.
126	Weight-lifting in women with breast cancer–related lymphedema	8/13/09	Breast cancer survivors with lymphedema (a common postsurgical complication) are commonly told to limit the use of the affected arm. This randomized trial showed that weight-lifting actually improves the symptoms of lymphedema (discussed in chapter 15).

	STUDY	DATE OF PUBLICATION	SUMMARY
127	Intensity of continuous renal-replacement therapy in critically ill patients	10/22/09	Prior to this study there had been a widespread increase in the use of higher-intensity continuous renal-replacement therapy among critically ill patients. This large, multicenter, randomized controlled trial of intensity of renal support showed that this practice was not justified.
128	Revascularization versus medical therapy for renal-artery stenosis	11/12/09	Renal artery stenosis is associated with hypertension and kidney disease, but it is unclear whether the relationship is causal. Despite this uncertainty, 16 percent of patients with newly diagnosed atherosclerotic narrowing of the renal artery and hypertension were treated for this narrowing. This large randomized trial found substantial risks but no evidence of benefit from this treatment.
129	A trial of darbepoetin alfa in type 2 diabetes and chronic kidney disease	11/19/09	Similar to study 80, this trial showed that the use of erythropoesis-stimulating agents among patients with anemia and chronic kidney disease did not reduce the risk of death, cardiovascular events, or renal events. It did show that the treatment was associated with an increased risk of stroke.
130	Extended-release niacin or ezetimibe and carotid intima-media thickness	11/26/09	Similar to study 106, this trial further undermined the purported benefit of ezetimibe with respect to cardiovascular risk.
131	Preoperative biliary drainage for cancer of the head of the pancreas	1/14/10	This study addressed a procedure to relieve jaundice prior to surgery in patients with pancreatic cancer. This multicenter, randomized trial found that the procedure, preoperative biliary drainage, increases the rate of serious complications without a mortality benefit.

STUDY	DATE OF PUBLICATION	SUMMARY
132 Outcomes after internal versus external tocodynamometry for monitoring labor	1/28/10	Recommendations existed regarding use of internal tocodynamometry—a means of monitoring uterine contractions—during cases of induction or augmentation of labor. This multicenter, randomized trial found that internal tocodynamometry did not reduce the rate of operative deliveries, adverse neonatal outcomes, analgesia use, antibiotics use, or time to delivery.
133 Comparison of dopamine and norepinephrine in the treatment of shock	3/4/10	This study compared the use of two medications commonly used to support the blood pressure in critically ill patients and found one to be clearly superior.
134 Lenient versus strict rate control in patients with atrial fibrillation	4/15/10	A challenge in treating patients with atrial fibrillation is controlling their heart rates. Guidelines recommended strict rate control (resting heart rate fewer than 80 beats per minute and exercise heart rate fewer than 110 beats per minute). This study found that more lenient rate control was not inferior to strict rate control (and was much easier to achieve).
135 Effects of combination lipid therapy in type 2 diabetes mellitus	4/29/10	Fibrates, which are cholesterol-lowering medications, are commonly combined with statins to treat high cholesterol. This study demonstrates that a combination of a statin and a fibrate was not superior to therapy with a statin alone.

STUDY	DATE OF PUBLICATION	SUMMARY
136 Effects of intensive blood-pressure control in type 2 diabetes mellitus	4/29/10	Guidelines recommended strict blood-pressure control in patients with diabetes. This study partially reversed these recommendations by showing that strict control did not differ from the standard control with respect to the study's primary outcome of nonfatal myocardial infarction, nonfatal stroke, or cardiovascular death. Intensive treatment did lower the stroke risk in intensively treated patients (though the absolute benefit was small and was associated with more adverse events).
137 Aspirin plus heparin or aspirin alone in women with recurrent miscarriage	4/29/10	This study evaluated the common practice of using antiplatelet and anticoagulation therapy during pregnancy in women with unexplained, recurrent miscarriages. The large multicenter study, which randomized these women to aspirin plus heparin, aspirin alone, or placebo, failed to demonstrate a benefit in live-birth rate with aspirin plus heparin or aspirin alone.
138 Quality indicators for colonoscopy and the risk of interval cancer	5/13/10	Professional societies advocated cecal intubation as a quality-indicator for colonoscopy. This large, retrospective study failed to demonstrate that cecal intubation was a predictor of interval colon cancer.

	STUDY	DATE OF PUBLICATION	SUMMARY
139	Long-term outcome of open or endovascular repair of abdominal aortic aneurysm	5/20/10	Recently, endovascular repair of abdominal aortic aneurysms has become popular because this approach improves perioperative survival over conventional open repair. This randomized, controlled trial showed similar survival rates between endovascular and open repairs but higher re-intervention rates for endovascular repair.
140	A randomized trial of treatment for acute anterior cruciate ligament tears	7/22/10	This study, discussed in chapter 2, randomized young, active adults to structured rehabilitation plus early ACL reconstructive surgery or structured rehabilitation with delayed ACL reconstruction. The results suggest that more than half of all surgical reconstructions can be reasonably avoided.
141	CPR with chest compression alone or with rescue breathing	7/29/10	Studies 141 and 142 test the nearly half-century-old assumption that chest compression and rescue breathing are critical parts of CPR. These trials showed no benefit from rescue breathing when added to chest compression.
142	Compression-only CPR or standard CPR in out-of-hospital cardiac arrest	7/29/10	See study 141.

	STUDY	DATE OF PUBLICATION	SUMMARY
143	Suicide-related events in patients treated with antiepileptic drugs	8/5/10	This represents a complicated reversal where a practice based on inadequate data was reversed by a study providing only slightly less inadequate data. In 2008 there was an FDA warning regarding the risk of suicidality associated with antiepileptic drugs. This case-control analysis showed that treatment with antiepileptic drugs did not increase the risk of suicide-related events in patients with epilepsy but did increase the risk among patients with depression and among those without epilepsy, depression, or bipolar disorder.
144	A randomized, controlled trial of early versus late initiation of dialysis	8/12/10	This trial suggested that initiating dialysis early, as widely recommended, is actually no better than a later initiation.
145	Gentamicin-collagen sponge for infection prophylaxis in colorectal surgery	9/9/10	The gentamicin-collagen sponge has been approved for use in numerous countries and used in millions of patients worldwide since 1985. Its use was based primarily on a single-center, randomized trial. This large, multicenter trial showed that the gentamicin-collagen sponge actually resulted in significantly more surgical-site infections, more visits to the emergency room or surgical office, and more hospitalizations for infection.
146	Effects of CYP2C19 genotype on outcomes of clopidogrel treatment	10/28/10	This study addressed the effectiveness of the blood-thinner clopidogrel in patients who metabolize drugs normally or more slowly. Contrary to previous understanding (and related practice), the present study showed that the safety and efficacy of clopidogrel is consistent, regardless of the rate of metabolism.

REFERENCES

INTRODUCTION

Boden WE, O'Rourke RA, Teo KK, et al., Optimal medical therapy with or without PCI for stable coronary disease. N Engl J Med. 2007;356:1503–1516.

Grodstein F, Stampfer MJ, Manson JE, et al. Postmenopausal estrogen and progestin use and the risk of cardiovascular disease. N Engl J Med. 1996;335:453–461.

Hulley S, Grady D, Bush T, et al. Randomized trial of estrogen plus progestin for secondary prevention of coronary heart disease in postmenopausal women. Heart and Estrogen/progestin Replacement Study (HERS) Research Group. JAMA. 1998;280:605–613.

McKinlay JB. From "promising report" to "standard procedure": Seven stages in the career of a medical innovation. Milbank Memorial Fund Quarterly. 1981;59:374–411.

1. WHAT IS MEDICAL REVERSAL?

Boden WE, O'Rourke RA, Teo KK, et al. Optimal medical therapy with or without PCI for stable coronary disease. N Engl J Med. 2007;356:1503–1516.

Buchbinder R, Osborne RH, Ebeling PR, et al. A randomized trial of vertebroplasty for painful osteoporotic vertebral fractures. N Engl J Med. 2009;361:557–568.

Carlberg B, Samuelsson O, Lindholm LH. Atenolol in hypertension: Is it a wise choice? Lancet. 2004;364:1684–1689.

Dahlof B, Devereux RB, Kjeldsen SE, et al. Cardiovascular morbidity and mortality in the Losartan Intervention For Endpoint reduction in hypertension study (LIFE): A randomised trial against atenolol. Lancet. 2002;359:995–1003.

Kallmes DF, Comstock BA, Heagerty PJ, et al. A randomized trial of vertebroplasty for osteoporotic spinal fractures. N Engl J Med. 2009;361:569–579.

Moss SM, Cuckle H, Evans A, Johns L, Waller M, Bobrow L. Effect of mammographic screening from age 40 years on breast cancer mortality at 10 years' follow-up: A randomised controlled trial. Lancet. 2006;368:2053–2060.

Parker ED, Margolis KL, Trower NK, et al. Comparative effectiveness of 2 β-blockers in hypertensive patients. Arch Intern Med. 2012;172(18):1406–1412.

2. SUBJECTIVE OUTCOMES

Beecher HK. Surgery as placebo: A quantitative study of bias. JAMA. 1961 Jul 1;176:1102–1107.

Cobb LA, Thomas GI, Dillard DH, et al. An evaluation of internal-mammary-artery ligation by a double-blind technic. N Engl J Med. 1959;260:1115–1118.

Frobell RB, Roos EM, Roos HP, et al. A randomized trial of treatment for acute anterior cruciate ligament tears. N Engl J Med. 2010;363:331–342.

Hróbjartsson A, Gøtzsche PC. Placebo interventions for all clinical conditions. Cochrane Database Syst Rev. 2010 Jan 20;(1):CD003974. doi: 10.1002/14651858.CD003974.pub3.

Kaptchuk TJ, Friedlander E, Kelley JM, et al. Placebos without deception: A randomized controlled trial in irritable bowel syndrome. PLOS One. 2010:5:e15591.

Kaptchuk TJ. The placebo effect in alternative medicine: Can the performance of a healing ritual have clinical significance. Ann Intern Med. 2002;136:817–825.

Katz JN, Brophy RH, Chaisson CE, et al. Surgery versus physical therapy for a meniscal tear and osteoarthritis. N Engl J Med. 2013;368:1675–1684.

Levine JD, Gordon NC, Fields HL. The mechanism of placebo analgesia. Lancet. 1978;312:654–657.

Podolsky S. Quintessential Beecher: Surgery as placebo: A quantitative study of bias. JAMA. 1961;176:1102–1107.

Redberg RF. Sham controls in medical device trials. N Engl J Med. 2014;371:892–893.

Rothberg MB, Sivalingam SK, Ashraf J, et al. Patients' and cardiologists' perceptions of the benefits of percutaneous coronary intervention for stable coronary disease. Ann Intern Med. 2010;153:307–313.

Sihvonen R, Paavola M, Malmivaara A, et al. Arthroscopic partial meniscectomy versus sham surgery for a degenerative meniscal tear. N Engl J Med. 2013;369:2515–2524.

Tricoci P, Allen JM, Kramer JM, et al. Scientific evidence underlying the ACC/AHA clinical practice guidelines. JAMA. 2009;301:831–841.

Wechsler ME, Kelley JM, Boyd IOE, et al. Active albuterol or placebo, sham acupuncture, or no intervention in asthma. N Engl J Med. 2011;365:119–126.

Weintraub WS, Spertus JA, Kolm P, et al. Effect of PCI on quality of life in patients with stable coronary disease. N Engl J Med. 2008;359:677–687.

Weisse AB. Saving lives, not sacrificing them: The inevitable clash between medical research and the protection of medical subjects. Bayl Univ Med Cent Proc. 2013;26: 306–310.

3. SURROGATE OUTCOMES

The ACCORD Study Group. Effects of combination lipid therapy in type 2 diabetes mellitus. N Engl J Med. 2010;362:1563–1574.

The Action to Control Cardiovascular Risk in Diabetes Study Group. Effects of intensive glucose lowering in type 2 diabetes. N Engl J Med. 2008;358:2545–2559.

The AIM-HIGH Investigators. Niacin in patients with low HDL cholesterol levels receiving intensive statin therapy. N Engl J Med. 2011;365:2255–2267.

Dickler M, Cobleigh M, Perez EA, et al. Paclitaxel plus bevacizumab versus paclitaxel alone for metastatic breast cancer. N Engl J Med. 2007;357:2666–2676.

Hemkens L, Contopoulos-Ioannidis DG, Ioannidis JPA. Concordance of effects of medical interventions on hospital admission and readmission rates with effects on mortality. CMAJ. 2013;185:E827–837.

Miller K, Wang M, Gralow J, et al. The ADVANCE collaborative group. Intensive blood glucose control and vascular outcomes in patients with type 2 diabetes. N Engl J Med. 2008;358:2560–2572.

Thiele H, Zeymer U, Neumann FJ, et al. Intraaortic balloon support for myocardial infarction with cardiogenic shock. N Engl J Med. 2012;367:1287–1296.

4. SCREENING TESTS

Aberle DR, Adams AM, Berg CD, et al. Reduced lung-cancer mortality with low-dose computed tomographic screening. N Engl J Med. 2011;365:395–409.

Atkin WS, Edwards R, Kralj-Hans I, et al. Once-only flexible sigmoidoscopy screening in prevention of colorectal cancer: A multicentre randomised controlled trial. Lancet. 2010;375:1624–1633.

Bleyer A, Welch HG. Effect of three decades of screening mammography on breast-cancer incidence. N Engl J Med. 2012;367:1998–2005.

Esserman L, Shieh Y, Thompson I. Rethinking screening for breast cancer and prostate cancer. JAMA. 2009;302:1685–1692.

Fang F, Keating NL, Mucci LA, et al. Immediate risk of suicide and cardiovascular death after a prostate cancer diagnosis: Cohort study in the United States. J Natl Cancer Inst. 2010;102:307–314.

Löwy I. Preventative Strikes: Women, Precancer, and Prophylactic Surgery. Baltimore: Johns Hopkins University Press; 2010.

Miller A, Wall C, Baines CJ, et al. Twenty five year follow-up for breast cancer incidence and mortality of the Canadian National Breast Screening Study: Randomised screening trial. BMJ. 2014;348:g366.

Moss SM, Cuckle H, Evans A, Johns L, Waller M, Bobrow L. Effect of mammographic screening from age 40 years on breast cancer mortality at 10 years' follow-up: A randomised controlled trial. Lancet. 2006;368:2053–2060.

Schröder FH, Hugosson J, Roobol MJ, et al. Screening and prostate-cancer mortality in a randomized European study. N Engl J Med. 2009;360:1320–1328.

Schröder FH, Hugosson J, Roobol MJ, et al. Screening and prostate cancer mortality: Results of the European Randomised Study of Screening for Prostate Cancer (ERSPC) at 13 years of follow-up. Lancet. 2014;384:2027–2035.

Shaukat A, Mongin SJ, Geisser MS, et al. Long-term mortality after screening for colorectal cancer. N Engl J Med. 2013;369:1106–1114.

Welch HG. Overdiagnosis in cancer. J Natl Cancer Inst. 2010;102:605–613.

Welch HG, Frankel BA. Likelihood that a woman with screen-detected breast cancer has had her "life saved" by that screening. Arch Intern Med. 2011;12:2043–2046.

5. SYSTEMS FAILURE

Abad C, Fearday A, Safdar N. Adverse effects of isolation in hospitalised patients: A systematic review. J Hosp Infect. 2010;76:97–102.

Climo MW, Yokoe DS, Warren DK, et al. Effect of daily chlorhexidine bathing on hospital-acquired infection. N Engl J Med. 2013;368:533–542.

Fung CH, Lim Y, Mattke S, et al. Systematic review: The evidence that publishing patient care performance data improves quality of care. Ann Intern Med. 2008;148:111–123.

Harris AD, Pineles L, Belton B, et al. Universal glove and gown use and acquisition of antibiotic-resistant bacteria in the ICU: A randomized trial. JAMA. 2013;310:1571–1580.

Huskins WC, Huckabee CM, O'Grady NP, et al. Intervention to reduce transmission of resistant bacteria in intensive care. N Engl J Med. 2011;364:1407–1418.

Ioannidis J, Prasad V. Evaluating health system processes with randomized controlled trials. JAMA Intern Med. 2013;173:1279–1280.

Krumholz HM, Bradley EH, Nallamothu BK, et al. A campaign to improve the timeliness of primary percutaneous coronary intervention—door-to-balloon: An alliance for quality. JACC Cardiovasc Interv. 2008;1:97–104.

Marsteller JA, Sexton JB, Hsu YJ, et al. A multicenter, phased, cluster-randomized controlled trial to reduce central line–associated bloodstream infections in intensive care units. Crit Care Med. 2012;40:2933–2939.

Menees DS, Peterson ED, Wang Y, et al. Door-to-balloon time and mortality among patients undergoing primary PCI. N Engl J Med. 2013;369:901–909.

MERIT study investigators. Introduction of the medical emergency team (MET) system: A cluster-randomised controlled trial. Lancet. 2005;365:2091–2097.

Naylor MD, Brooten D, Campbell R, et al. Comprehensive discharge planning and home follow-up of hospitalized elders: A randomized clinical trial. JAMA. 1999;281:613–620.

NICE-SUGAR study investigators. Intensive versus conventional glucose control in critically ill patients. N Engl J Med. 2009;360:1283–1297.

Van den Berghe G, Wilmer A, Hermans G, et al. Intensive insulin therapy in the medical ICU. N Engl J Med. 2006;354:449–461.

Van den Berghe G, Wouters P, Weekers F, et al. Intensive insulin therapy in critically ill patients. N Engl J Med. 2001;345:1359–1367.

Wachter RM, Flanders SA, Fee C, et al. Public reporting of antibiotic timing in patients with pneumonia: Lessons from a flawed performance measure. Ann Intern Med. 2008;149:29–32.

6. FINDING FLAWED THERAPIES ON OUR OWN

Barnes PM, Bloom B, Nahin RL. Complementary and alternative medicine use among adults and children: United States, 2007. Natl Health Stat Report. 2008;12:1–23.

Bolland MJ, Avenell A, Baron JA, et al. Effect of calcium supplements on risk of myocardial infarction and cardiovascular events: Meta-analysis. BMJ. 2010;341:c3691.

Bolland MJ, Grey A, Avenell A, et al. Calcium supplements with or without vitamin D and risk of cardiovascular events: Reanalysis of the Women's Health Initiative limited access dataset and meta-analysis. BMJ. 2011;342:d2040.

Chung M, Lee J, Terasawa T, et al. Vitamin D with or without calcium supplementation for prevention of cancer and fractures: An updated meta-analysis for the U.S. Preventive Services Task Force. Ann Intern Med. 2011;155:827–838.

Clegg DO, Reda DJ, Harris CL, et al. Glucosamine, chondroitin sulfate, and the two in combination for painful knee osteoarthritis. N Engl J Med. 2006;354:795–808.

Ernst E, Lee MS, Choi TY. Acupuncture: Does it alleviate pain and are there serious risks? A review of reviews. Pain. 2011;152:755–764.

Estruch R, Ros E, Salas-Salvadó J, et al. Primary prevention of cardiovascular disease with a Mediterranean diet. N Engl J Med. 2013;368:1279–1290.

Fortmann SP, Burda BU, Senger CA, et al. Vitamin and mineral supplements in the primary prevention of cardiovascular disease and cancer: An updated systematic evidence review for the U.S. Preventive Services Task Force. Ann Intern Med. 2013;159:824–834.

Guallar E, Stranges S, Mulrow C. Enough is enough: Stop wasting money on vitamin and mineral supplements. Ann Intern Med. 2013;159:850–851.

Karsch-Völk M, Barrett B, Kiefer D, et al. Echinacea for preventing and treating the common cold. Cochrane Database Syst Rev. 2014 Feb 20.

Neuhouser M L, Wassertheil-Smoller S, Thomson C. Multivitamin use and risk of cancer and cardiovascular disease in the Women's Health Initiative cohorts. Arch Intern Med. 2009;169:294–304.

Schoenfeld JD, Ioannidis JP. Is everything we eat associated with cancer? A systematic cookbook review. Am J Clin Nutr. 2013;97:127–134.

Turner RB, Bauer R, Woelkart K, et al. An evaluation of echinacea angustifolia in experimental rhinovirus infections. N Engl J Med. 2005;353:341–348.

Wandel S, Jüni P, Tendal B, et al. Effects of glucosamine, chondroitin, or placebo in patients with osteoarthritis of hip or knee: Network meta-analysis. BMJ. 2010;341:c4675.

7. THE FREQUENCY OF MEDICAL REVERSAL

Elshaug A, Watt A, Mundy L, Willis CD. Over 150 potentially low-value health care practices: An Australian study. Med J Aust. 2012;197(10):556–560.

Ioannidis JA. Contradicted and initially stronger effects in highly cited clinical research. JAMA. 2005;294(2):218–228.

Prasad V, Gall V, Cifu A. The frequency of medical reversal. Arch Intern Med. 2011;171(18):1675–1676.

Prasad V, Vandross A, Toomey C, et al. A decade of reversal: An analysis of 146 contradicted medical practices. Mayo Clin Proc. 2013;88(8):790–798.

8. THE HARMS OF MEDICAL REVERSAL

Cannon CP, Braunwald E, McCabe CH, et al. Intensive versus moderate lipid lowering with statins after acute coronary syndromes. N Engl J Med. 2004;350:1495–1504.

Chimowitz MI, Lynn MJ, Derdeyn CP, et al. Stenting versus aggressive medical therapy for intracranial arterial stenosis. N Engl J Med. 2011;365:993–1003.

Hartzband P, Groopman J. There is more to life than death. N Engl J Med. 2012;367:987–989.

Kjekshus J, Apatrei E, Barrios V, et al. Rosuvastatin in older patients with systolic heart failure. N Engl J Med. 2007;357:2248–2261.

Prasad V, Cifu A. Medical reversal: Why we must raise the bar before adopting new technologies. Yale J Biol Med. 2011;84:471–478.

Reinberg S. Study: "Brain stents" for stroke patients do more harm than good. USA Today. www.usatoday.com/news/health/story/health/story/2011-09-08/Study-Brain-stents-for-stroke-patients-do-more-harm-than-good/50321642/1.

Roman B, Asch DA, Faded promises: The challenge of deadopting low-value care. Ann Intern Med. 2014;161:149–150.

Siontis GC, Tatsioni A, Katritsis DG, Ioannidis JP. Persistent reservations against contradicted percutaneous coronary intervention indications: Citation content analysis. Am Heart J. 2009;157:695–701.

Smith CM. Origin and uses of primum non nocere—above all, do no harm! J Clin Pharmacol. 2005;45:371–377.

Tatsioni A, Bonitsis NG, Ioannidis JA. Persistence of contradicted claims in the literature. JAMA. 2007;298:2517–2526.

Weiss M. Lives will be lost with proposed changes to mammography guidelines. Fox News. www.foxnews.com/opinion/2009/11/17/new-breast-cancer-guidelines-mammograms-guidelines-lives-lost/#ixzz27VJvcTii.

9. A PRIMER ON EVIDENCE-BASED MEDICINE

Byer DB, Simon RM, Fridewald WT, et al. Randomized clinical trials: Perspectives on some recent ideas. N Engl J Med. 1976;296:74–80.

Cnattingius S, Signorello LB, Annerén G, et al. Caffeine intake and the risk of first trimester spontaneous abortion. N Engl J Med. 2000;343:1839–1845.

Godtfredsen NS, Prescott E, Osler M. Effect of smoking reduction on lung cancer risk. JAMA. 2005;294:1505–1510.

Grodstein F, Stampfer MJ, Manson JE, et al. Postmenopausal estrogen and progestin use and the risk of cardiovascular disease. N Engl J Med. 1996;335:453–461.

Ioannidis JA, Haidich A, Pappa M, et al. Comparison of evidence of treatment effects in randomized and nonrandomized studies. JAMA. 2001;286:821–830.

Scandinavian Simvastatin Survival Study Group. Randomized trial of cholesterol lowering in 4444 patients with coronary heart disease: The Scandinavian Simvastatin Survival Study (4S). Lancet. 1994;344:1383–1389.

Stampfer MJ, Colditz GA, Willett WC, et al. Postmenopausal estrogen therapy and cardiovascular disease: Ten-year follow-up from the nurses' health study. N Engl J Med. 1999;325:756–762.

Streptomycin in Tuberculosis Trials Committee. Streptomycin treatment of pulmonary tuberculosis. BMJ. 1948;2:769.

10. WHAT REALLY MADE YOU BETTER

Bassler D, Briel M, Montori VM, et al. Stopping randomized trials early for benefit and estimation of treatment effects systematic review and meta-regression analysis. JAMA. 2010;303:1180–1187.

Borzak S, Ridker PM. Discordance between meta-analyses and large-scale randomized, controlled trials: Examples from the management of acute myocardial infarction. Ann Intern Med. 1995;123:873–877.

Gilbert AT, Petersen BW, Recuenco S, et al. Evidence of rabies virus exposure among humans in the Peruvian Amazon. Am J Trop Med Hyg. 2012;87:206–215.

Goodman S. Toward evidence-based medical statistics. 1: The P value fallacy. Ann Intern Med. 1999;130:995–1004.

Ioannidis JPA. Why most published research findings are false. PLOS. 2005;2:e124.

LeLorier J, Grégoire G, Benhaddad A, et al. Discrepancies between meta-analyses and subsequent large randomized, controlled trials. N Engl J Med. 1997;337:536–542.

Pereira TV, Horwitz RI, Ioannidis JPA. Empirical evaluation of very large treatment effects of medical interventions. JAMA. 2012;308:1676–1684.

Smith CS, Pell JP. Parachute use to prevent death and major trauma related to gravitational challenge: Systematic review of randomised controlled trials. BMJ. 2003;327:1459.

Varadhan KK, Neal KR, Lobo DN. Safety and efficacy of antibiotics compared with appendectomy for treatment of uncomplicated acute appendicitis: Meta-analysis of randomised controlled trials. BMJ. 2012;344:e2156.

Willoughby RE Jr, Tieves KS, et al. Survival after treatment of rabies with induction of coma. N Engl J Med. 2005;352:2508-2514.

Worrall J. Why there's no cause to randomize. Br J Philos Sci. 2007;58:451–488.

11. SCIENTIFIC PROGRESS, REVOLUTION, AND MEDICAL REVERSAL

Arnowitz RA. Making Sense of Illness: Science, Society, and Disease. Cambridge: Cambridge University Press; 1998.

Jones DS. Broken Hearts: The Tangled History of Cardiac Care. Baltimore, MD: Johns Hopkins University Press; 2013.

Kahn IA, Mehta NJ. Initial historical descriptions of the angina pectoris. J Emerg Med. 2002;22:295–298.

Kuhn T. The Structure of Scientific Revolutions. 3rd ed. Chicago, IL: University of Chicago Press; 1996.

Kureshi F, Jones PG, Buchanan DM, et al. Variation in patients' perceptions of elective percutaneous coronary intervention in stable coronary artery disease: Cross sectional study. BMJ. 2014;349:g5309.

Nabel, EG, Braunwald E. A tale of coronary artery disease and myocardial infarction. N Engl J Med. 2012;366:54–63.

12. SOURCES OF FLAWED DATA

Angell M. The Truth about Drug Companies: How They Deceive Us and What to Do about It. New York, NY. Random House; 2004.

Dhruva SS, Bero LA, Redberg RF. Strength of study evidence examined by the FDA in premarket approval of cardiovascular devices. JAMA. 2009;302:2679–2685.

Eichacker PQ, Natanson C, Danner RL. Surviving sepsis—practice guidelines, marketing campaigns, and Eli Lilly. N Engl J Med. 2006;355:1640–1642.

Jefferson T, Jones M, Doshi P, et al. Oseltamivir for influenza in adults and children: Systematic review of clinical study reports and summary of regulatory comments. BMJ. 2014;348:2545.

Kesselheim AS, Robertson CT, Myers JA, et al. A randomized study of how physicians interpret research funding disclosures. N Engl J Med. 2012;367:1119–1127.

Kumar K, Taylor RS, Jacques L. The effects of spinal cord stimulation in neuropathic pain are sustained: A 24-month follow-up of the prospective randomized controlled multicenter trial of the effectiveness of spinal cord stimulation. Neurosurgery. 2008;63:762–770.

Lexchin J, Bero LA, Djulbegovic B, et al. Pharmaceutical industry sponsorship and research outcome and quality: Systematic review. BMJ. 2003;326:1167.

Lundh A, Sismondo S, Lexchin J, et al. Industry sponsorship and research outcome. Cochrane Library. www.thecochranelibrary.com/details/file/3994131/MR000033.html.

Muthuri SG, Venkatesan S, Myles PR, et al. Effectiveness of neuraminidase inhibitors in reducing mortality in patients admitted to hospital with influenza A H1N1pdm09 virus infection: A meta-analysis of individual participant data. *Lancet Respir Med.* 2014;2:395–404.

Pencina MJ, Navar-Boggan AM, D'Agostino RB, et al. Application of new cholesterol guidelines to a population-based sample. N Engl J Med. 2014;370:1422–1431.

Prasad V. Statins, primary prevention, overall mortality. Ann Intern Med. 2014;160:867–869.

Prasad V, Massey PR, Fojo T. Oral anticancer drugs: How limited dosing options and dose reductions may affect outcomes in comparative trials and efficacy in patients. J Clin Oncol. 2014;32:1620–1629.

Rome BN, Kramer DB, Kesselheim AS. FDA approval of cardiac implantable electronic devices via original and supplement premarket approval pathways, 1979–2012. JAMA. 2009;302:2679–2685.

13. WHY ARE WE SO ATTRACTED TO FLAWED THERAPIES?

Carman KL, Maurer M, Yegian JM, et al. Evidence that consumers are skeptical about evidence-based health care. Health Aff. 2010:29;1400–1406.

Donohue JM, Cevasco M, Rosenthal MB. A decade of direct-to-consumer advertising of prescription drugs. N Engl J Med. 2007;357:673–681.

Hu FB, Li TY, Colditz GA, et al. Television watching and other sedentary behaviors in relation to risk of obesity and type 2 diabetes mellitus in women. JAMA. 2003;289:1785–1791.

Huedo-Medina TB, Kirsch I, Middlemass J, et al. Effectiveness of non-benzodiazepine hypnotics in treatment of adult insomnia: Meta-analysis of data submitted to the Food and Drug Administration. BMJ. 2012;345:e8343.

Masters RK, Reither EN, Powers DA, et al. The impact of obesity on US mortality levels: The importance of age and cohort factors in population estimates. Am J Public Health. 2013;103:1895–1901.

Mitchell JM. Urologists' use of intensity-modulated radiation therapy for prostate cancer. N Engl J Med. 2013;369:1629–1637.

Kravitz RL, Epstein RM, et al. Influence of patients' requests for direct-to-consumer advertised antidepressants: A randomized controlled trial. JAMA. 2005;293:1995–2002.

Slutsky AS. Improving outcomes in critically ill patients: The seduction of physiology. JAMA. 2009;302:2030–2032.

14. MEDICAL EDUCATION

Prasad V. Beyond storytelling in medicine: An encounter based curriculum. Acad Med. 2010;85:794–798.

Prasad V, Cifu A. A medical burden of proof: Towards a new physician ethic. BioSocieties. 2012;7:72–87.

15. ACADEMIC MEDICINE

Brett AS. Coronary assessment before noncardiac surgery: Current strategies are flawed. Circulation. 2008;117:3145–3151.

Schmitz KH, Ahmed RL, Troxel A, et al. Weight lifting in women with breast-cancer-related lymphedema. N Engl J Med. 2009;361:664–673.

16. REFORMING THE SYSTEM

Bleyer AW, Tejada H, Murphy SB, et al. National cancer clinical trials: Children have equal access; adolescents do not. J Adolesc Health. 1997;21:366–373.

Downs-Canner S, Shaw P. A comparison of clinical trial enrollment between adolescent and young adult (AYA) oncology patients treated at affiliated adult and pediatric oncology centers. J Pediatr Hematol Oncol. 2009;31:927–929.

Dubner SJ. There's no such thing as a free appetizer: A new Freakonomics radio podcast. Freakonomics. http://freakonomics.com/2014/06/19/theres-no-such-thing-as-a-free-appetizer-a-new-freakonomics-radio-podcast/.

Emanuel EJ, Schnipper LE, Kamin DY, et al. The costs of conducting clinical research. J Clin Oncol. 2003;21:4145–4150.

Lauer MS, D'Agostino RB. The randomized registry trial—the next disruptive technology in clinical research? N Engl J Med. 2013;369:1579–1581.

Prasad V, Cifu A. A medical burden of proof: Towards a new ethic. BioSocieties. 2012;7:72–87.

Prasad V, Rho J, Cifu A. The inferior vena cava filter: How could a medical device be so well accepted without any evidence of efficacy? JAMA Intern Med. 2013;173:493–494.

Sequist LV, Yang JC-H, Yamamoto N, et al. Phase III study of afatinib or cisplatin plus pemetrexed in patients with metastatic lung adenocarcinoma with EGFR mutations. J Clin Oncol. 2013;31:3327–3334.

Unger JM, Hershman DL, Albain KS, et al. Patient income level and cancer clinical trial participation. J Clin Oncol. 2013;31:536–542.

Weiss JP, Parsons LS, Every NR, et al. Does enrollment in a randomized clinical trial lead to a higher cost of routine care? Am Heart J. 2002;143:140–144.

Zhu AX, Kudo M, Assenat E, et al. Effect of everolimus on survival in advanced hepatocellular carcinoma after failure of sorafenib: The EVOLVE-1 randomized clinical trial. JAMA. 2014;312:57–67.

17. HOW NOT TO BECOME A VICTIM OF REVERSAL

Judson TJ, Detsky AS, Press MJ. Encouraging patients to ask questions: How to overcome "white-coat silence." JAMA. 2013;309:2325–2326.

18. BEYOND DOGMA

Grupp SA, Kalos M, Barrett D. Chimeric antigen receptor–modified t cells for acute lymphoid leukemia. N Engl J Med. 2013;368:1509–1518.

Pneumocystis Pneumonia—Los Angeles. MMWR. 1981;30:1–3.

Prasad V, Cheung M, Cifu A. Chest pain in the emergency department: The case against our current practice of routine noninvasive testing. Arch Intern Med. 2012;172:1506–1509.

Prasad V, Jorgenson J, Ioannidis JP, Cifu A. Observational studies often make clinical practice recommendations: An empirical evaluation of authors' attitudes. J Clin Epidemiol. 2013;66:361–366.

INDEX

VINAYAK K. PRASAD, MD, MPH, is a practicing hematologist-
oncologist and internal medicine physician. He completed his training
at the National Cancer Institute and the National Institutes of Health
in Bethesda, Maryland. He is an associate professor of medicine and public health at Oregon Health & Science University. Dr. Prasad's research
focuses on oncology drugs, health policy, evidence-based medicine, bias,
and medical reversal. He is the author of more than 90 peer-reviewed
articles in academic journals, including the *New England Journal of Medicine* and the *Journal of the American Medical Association.*

::

ADAM S. CIFU, MD, is a professor of medicine at the Pritzker School
of Medicine, University of Chicago. He is a practicing general internist
and teaches courses in clinical medicine and in reading and understanding the medical literature. He is the coauthor of a textbook on clinical
reasoning, *Symptom to Diagnosis: An Evidence-Based Guide,* which is now
in its third edition. He is a Master in the Academy of Distinguished Medical Educators at the University of Chicago.